IMAGES
of America

WESTBOROUGH
STATE HOSPITAL

On the Cover: Each year, the Westborough State Hospital marked both the Fourth of July and Labor Day with a field day celebration for staff and patients. Pictured is the 1947 Fourth of July field day held on the main lawn of the administration building. (Courtesy Westborough Public Library.)

IMAGES
of America

WESTBOROUGH
STATE HOSPITAL

Katherine Anderson
Introduction by Mimi Baird

ARCADIA
PUBLISHING

Copyright © 2019 by Katherine Anderson
ISBN 978-1-4671-0318-3

Published by Arcadia Publishing
Charleston, South Carolina

Printed in the United States of America

Library of Congress Control Number: 2018965130

For all general information, please contact Arcadia Publishing:
Telephone 843-853-2070
Fax 843-853-0044
E-mail sales@arcadiapublishing.com
For customer service and orders:
Toll-Free 1-888-313-2665

Visit us on the Internet at www.arcadiapublishing.com

CONTENTS

ACKNOWLEDGMENTS

As one of the last state hospitals to close in Massachusetts, the enduring legacy of Westborough State Hospital lives in the recent memory of the many men and women who lived and worked on the campus, as well as the patients who were treated there over the course of nearly 150 years.

This book would not have been possible without the help of former state representative Christine Canavan, current state representative Thomas Golden, and Anthony Vaver, local history librarian at the Westborough Public Library who welcomed me into his space and gave me access to an incredible collection of images. Equally, the Department of Mental Health with the assistance of the director of communication and community engagement Daniela Trammell and program coordinator Kristin Kulig were instrumental in bringing this book to life. Many thanks as well to historian and photographer Jon Maynard, who painstakingly digitized a number of images from the Department of Mental Health archive, many of which have not been shared with the public in years.

A great debt of thanks is also owed to local historian and former firefighter Phil Kittredge, who welcomed me into his home and shared his collection of Westborough history. His painstaking chronicle of Westborough town history has helped shape this book in so many ways.

To Mimi Baird, who has graciously shared the story of her father's time at Westborough and who has been an unflagging supporter of this project—I owe you a great debt of gratitude!

Finally, to the men and women who lived and worked at Westborough State Hospital, this history is a testament to the changing landscape of mental healthcare and the unflagging spirit of patients and staff alike.

INTRODUCTION

My father, Dr. Perry Baird, a prominent Boston physician, suffered from manic depressive psychosis. He was incarcerated in Westborough State Hospital multiple times in the 1940s, during the World War II years. Even though, as a child, I lived not far away in Chestnut Hill, I had no idea where he was. Back in those days, families kept untidy secrets to themselves and from their children. All I knew was that my father was "away."

Then, in 1991, I came across some information about my father, which started years of searching for clues as to why my father had disappeared from my life. One of my main sources of enlightenment became his Westborough medical records. I was fortunate to obtain these records just a few years before the enactment by the US Congress of HIPAA (Health Insurance Portability and Accountability Act) in 1996, which allows a patient his or her privacy when receiving medical treatment.

In February 1995, I decided to visit Westborough. On a clear winter day, I drove along Route 9 West from Boston, the same route the police would have followed as they delivered my father to the hospital. A half hour west of Route 495, I saw the hospital's sign and passed through a great stone gate. This was the place my father detested, and it remained much as he described in his memoir.

The hospital, at this time, resembled a small community college with its buildings huddled together on a hill surrounded by fields that no longer yield crops. Beyond these fields were dense woods with no visible signs of suburban housing. For a visitor traveling the long winding driveway, the entrance presented an elegant arrival to a place that, for many years, housed mentally ill patients. There was an abundance of tall majestic trees scattered among the six brick buildings including Codman and Talbot. During my father's time, Upper Codman was the floor reserved for the seriously ill and violent patients, while the bottom floor takes care of those whose behavior was relatively calm. Both Codman and Talbot were named after prominent Bostonians who contributed financial support to Westborough in the early 1900s. Most likely, family members and friends were treated there.

It was pretty well known that the care of mentally ill patients during World War II wasn't the optimum. In the spring of 1997, I was invited to give a talk about my father to the C. Everett Koop Institute at Dartmouth Hitchcock Medical Center/ Dartmouth Medical School. As a result of this presentation, I was then asked to give it again later that summer to Psychiatric Grand Rounds. When I finished, a distinguished gentleman sitting in the front row raised his hand. He was the greatly respected recently retired head of the Department of Psychiatry. On behalf of the specialty of psychiatry, he apologized to me for the treatment my father received while institutionalized during this time in our country's history. Everyone in the auditorium understood his statement, and a silence fell upon the attendees as they filed out of the room.

I continued to travel the long drive to the hospital, curving uphill, through vast lawns with remnants of snowbanks melting by the road. I had called ahead, so when I pulled up next to the refurbished Victorian administrative building, the staff was expecting me. This was the spot where my father had also arrived so many times, greeting doctors as if nothing unusual had occurred in the recent days of his life. A member of the staff directed me toward the Codman Building.

As described by my father, Codman was a two-story brick edifice complete with porches and a cupola. A young hospital worker showed me both floors of the building where occupational therapy now takes place. Patients, looking pale and ill at ease, were at work or walking the halls, some smoking or moving incessantly. The corridors on both floors were long and dark. The old walls were pained a drab gray. The small rooms that housed patients were now offices. The larger space, once wards and recreational areas, were unused or transformed as workspaces. I entered a large room with old oak tables and wondered if my father had sat there passing his endless and useless days. I looked across the lawns from a dusty window and wondered how many times he had looked through the same window. I saw a heavy metal staircase, reinforced with iron mesh, connecting the floors, and I wondered how many times my father's slippered feet had trod them. I felt like I was walking in his footsteps.

In one sizable room, now used for storage, I moved a sheet of plywood and found that it concealed a large tub, possibly used for the continuous bath treatments that my father endured. I wondered where my father had been when they applied the cold packs and straight-jackets. I recalled he had written about the filth of the toilets and how friends had told me he was so fastidious.

I wandered into the main living room of the top floor and looked around. Quite by accident, I glanced back toward the corridor I had just come through. The afternoon light flickered on the wall and floor, giving the perception of shimmering, transparent figures floating through the air. I had suddenly seen enough. I thanked my host and went outside into the fresh, cold air. I quickly got into my car and left the hospital grounds, free to leave, free of this place, and free to go on with my life.

Years later, in January 2016, I visited Westborough State Hospital again. This time, the buildings were in a state of complete disrepair. Mold, deteriorating interior walls, chunks of hanging plaster, disabled furniture, bird droppings, trash of every imaginable kind, and broken windows were evident. The manager of the grounds gave me a mask to wear, stating that these complexes were to be demolished in the near future. I visited both the Administration Building and Codman. The most searing visual was the following: on the landing of the steel staircase, leading from Upper Codman down to Lower Codman, was a window. Over the window was a summer screen. Embedded in the mesh was a dead pigeon. I couldn't help but recall my father's words as he was driven by the state police from his formal country club Sunday lunch, away from his friends and family, toward Westborough in February 1944: "I am caught, caught, caught."

Mimi Baird
author of *He Wanted the Moon: The Madness and Medical Genius of Dr. Perry Baird, and His Daughter's Quest to Know Him*

One

TRANSFORMATION

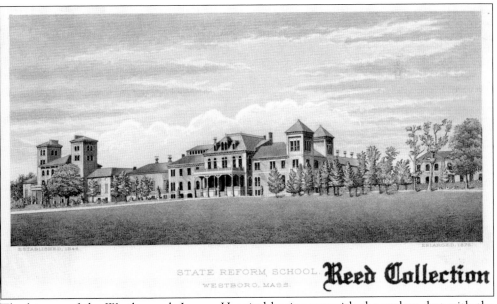

The history of the Westborough Insane Hospital begins not with the asylum, but with the Massachusetts State Reform School, the first state-operated reform school in the country. Designed by Elias Carter of Springfield and James Savage of Southborough, the school was built to house and rehabilitate 300 boys up to the age of 16. (Courtesy Phil Kittredge.)

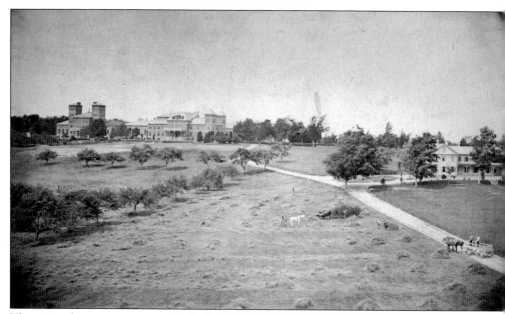

The original campus was comprised of 200 acres of farmland, which encompassed the farmstead of Lovett Peters, as well as land owned by the Rice family. The campus expanded from 275 acres in 1884 to nearly 600 acres in the early 1900s. The location offered ready access to roadways and railways. Later, the campus could be reached by Route 9 and the Worcester Turnpike. (Courtesy Westborough Public Library.)

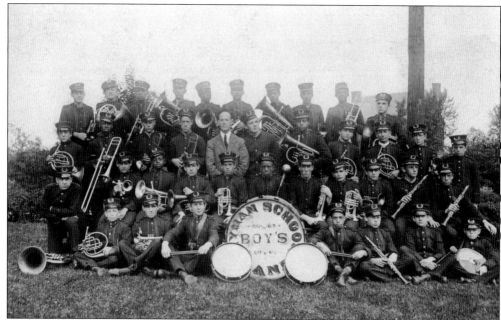

Later renamed for Boston mayor Theodore Lyman, the school's goal was the reform of young men who were considered "troublesome," though some would be sent to prison instead if it was decided they were incapable of returning to society. The school quickly outgrew its walls and expanded to nearly twice its size in 1852. The resulting building exists in nearly original form as the eastern end of Westborough State Hospital. (Courtesy Phil Kittredge.)

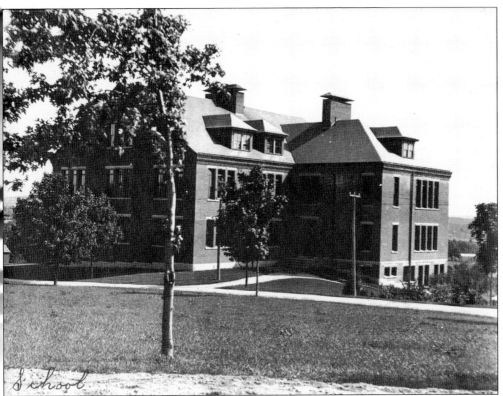

In 1885, the Massachusetts state legislature deemed the existing campus "unfit for reform school purposes due to its size" and approved the purchase of a new site for the Lyman School on Powder Hill on the western shore of Lake Chauncy. The school shifted from the original congregate model employed since its opening in 1848 to the dispersed system of organization with various smaller buildings arranged about the campus. (Courtesy Westborough State Hospital.)

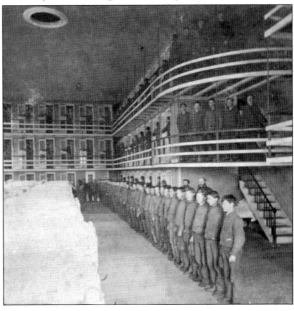

The buildings on the Lyman campus hadn't been kept up. Roofs were leaking, and the walls were found to be weak where the cells had been stripped. The first alterations to the reform school began on May 18, 1885, and the hospital intended to take in 400 patients. The first superintendent, N. Emmons Paine, said of the building, "It had guarded criminals. It must henceforth shelter the sick." (Courtesy Phil Kittredge.)

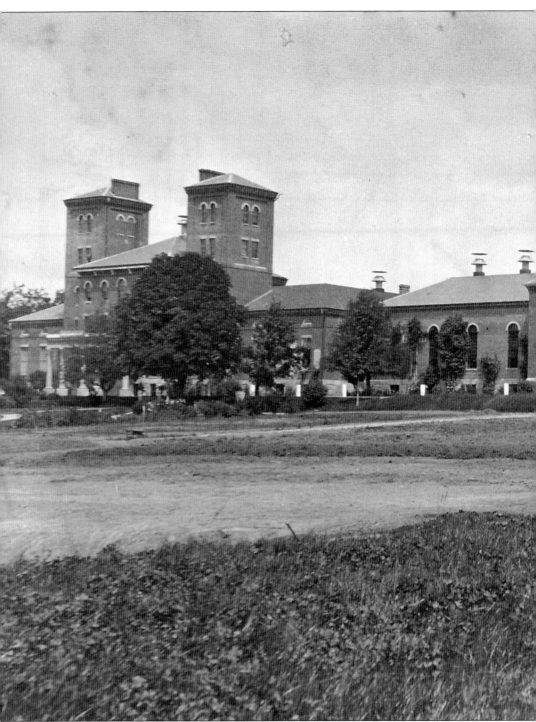

Most of the buildings that were original to the reform school were constructed between the time of its founding in 1848 and its closure in 1885. The main school building had been expanded and reconstructed a number of times, as had many of the outbuildings that no longer stand on the state hospital property. As can be seen in the next photograph, there was a large brick building

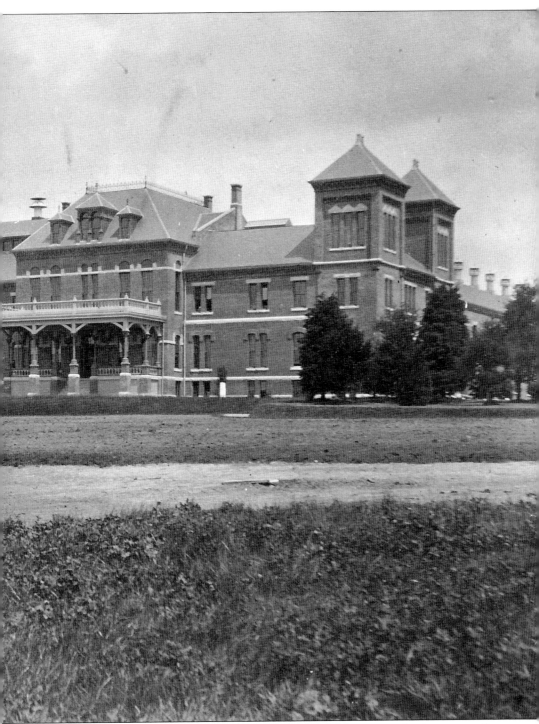

with bars on the windows that sat very near to the right side of the main school structure. By the time the reform school closed, this building was gone, along with much of the staff housing that had been provided for the officers of the school. The remainder of the former campus was left temporarily vacant. (Courtesy Phil Kittredge.)

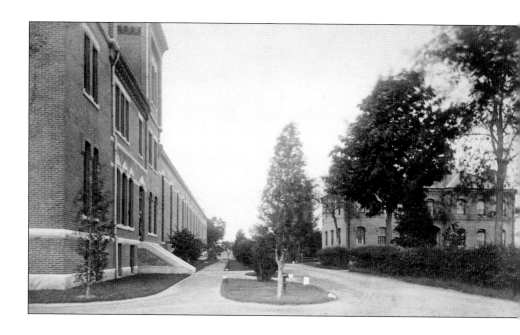

The reform school originally had ornate gardens and detailed landscaping in front of the main building. Unfortunately, this was lost sometime before the transition to an insane hospital. The gardens were likely tended by the boys who were sentenced to Lyman. Some things did survive however, such as the Lyman School's barns which were put to use by the hospital the moment they opened, allowing them to continue farming the land that had been worked by the inmates of the reform school. Those barns would later be destroyed and replaced by more modern barns that were demolished in the early 2000s. (Both, courtesy Phil Kittredge.)

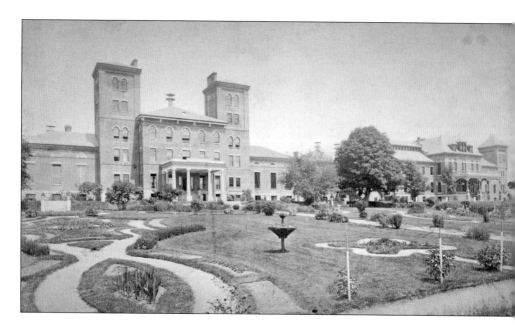

The state reform school property consisted of 164 acres with one large dorm that once housed up to five hundred boys and a number of cottages. There was an existing boiler house, cattle barn, piggery, icehouse, carriage houses, and a chair shop. It was decided that the property would no longer be used as a correction facility; instead, it would be converted into a hospital for the insane. (Courtesy Westborough Public Library.)

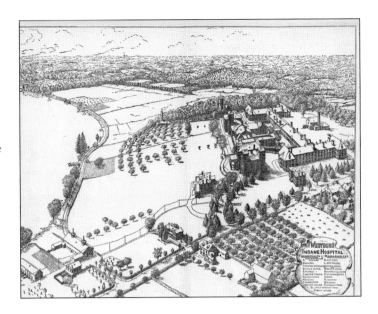

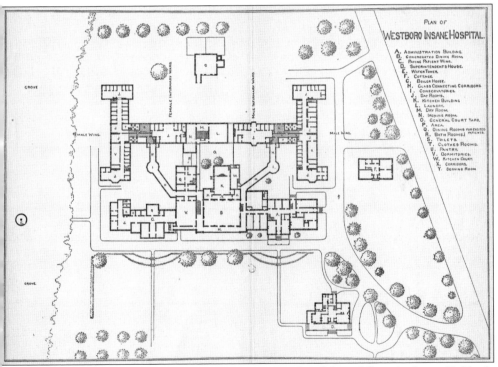

Westborough was the first asylum built in Massachusetts that did not follow the linear Kirkbride Plan, with a main administration building flanked by stepped-back wards. It was also one of the earliest examples of institutional adaptive reuse. Previous Massachusetts asylums were built on sites chosen specifically for the purpose of new construction. Westborough was created out of the recently renovated reform school and preserved its oldest extant building. There are two acceptable spellings of Westborough. Both were used interchangeably throughout the state hospital's history; therefore, both spellings are used in this book. (Courtesy Westborough State Hospital.)

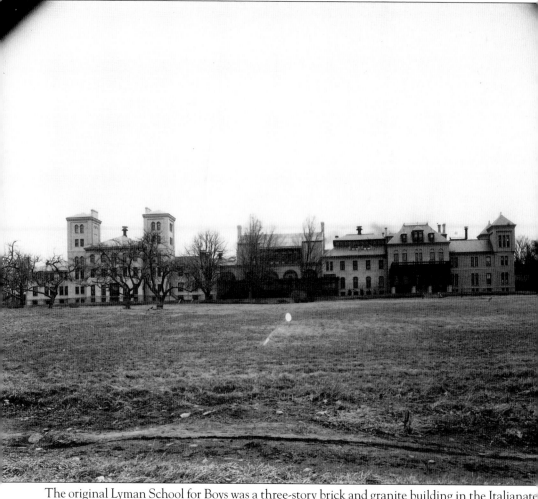

The original Lyman School for Boys was a three-story brick and granite building in the Italianate style. Within the walls were lodging rooms for the boys, storerooms, and a number of workshops to employ the boys. The lodging rooms were little more than cells, much like a modern jail, with open spaces on the floor for meals and other gatherings. In converting it for use as an asylum, Boston architect George Clough demolished the center of the building (which had been added in 1876) and replaced it with a gambrel roof section with a congregate dining hall on the first floor and a chapel on the second that had enormous windows offering views of both the lake and the farm. (Courtesy Phil Kittredge.)

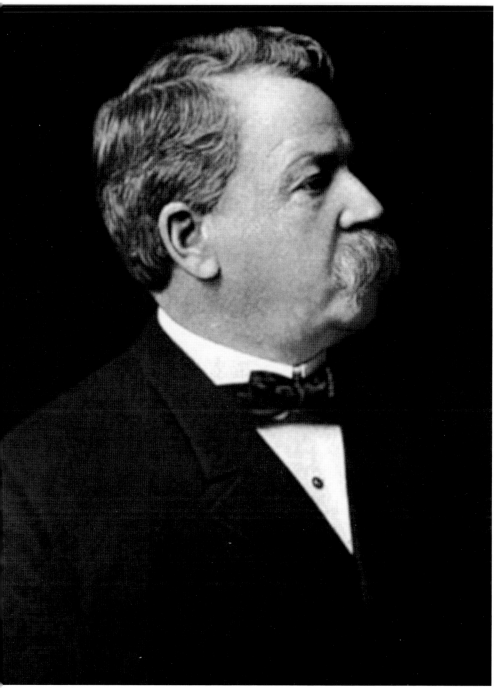

George Clough was fresh from a ten-year stint as Boston's first city architect when he was hired to complete two jobs simultaneously: first to reuse the old Lyman campus and then to design the new Lyman campus on the opposite shore of Lake Chauncy. The existing school was to be refitted for occupancy by 325 patients who would be transferred from the already overcrowded Kirkbrides. Boston landscape architect Joseph Curtis was hired to design the expansive grounds that swept down to the banks of Lake Chauncy. (Courtesy Massachusetts Biographical Society.)

Main Bldg.
Westboro Hospital

The outside walls and roof of the reform school were only altered in three places. Forty-foot sections were removed, and the old kitchen was "cleared away." The wards were added onto, and the first-floor chapel was converted into a dining hall, which allowed for a new one to be built above it that served not only as a chapel but also as a stage for performances, a shuffleboard court.

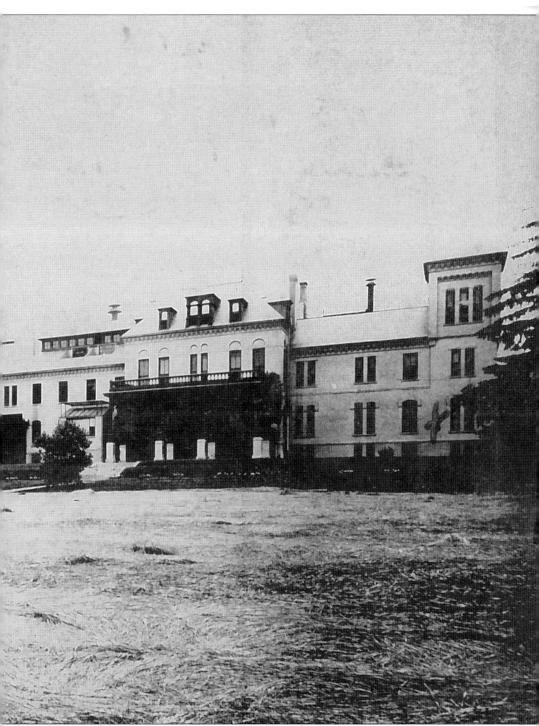

and a gymnasium. The old windows, many of them broken, were replaced, and new windows were cut to let in more light. The difference was slight but enough to brighten the interior. (Courtesy Westborough Public Library.)

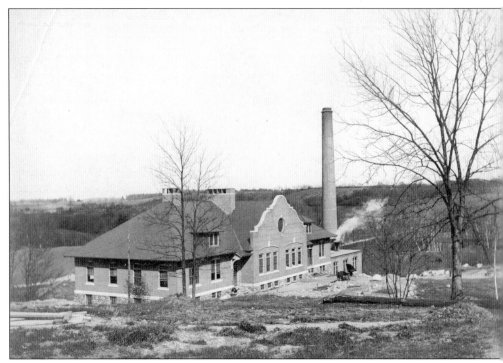

The original boiler plant, later the farm office, provided steam heat for the main hospital. The plant was built in 1886 as part of the campus-wide changes needed in order to expand the reform school and retrofit the buildings for hospital use. A number of radiators and pipes had already been removed during construction and would be repaired and made usable again. The trustees noted in their first annual report that the boiler "has of course to stand the test of a winter's use,' a fair consideration in New England, where winters could be quite difficult to weather. (Both courtesy Westborough Public Library.)

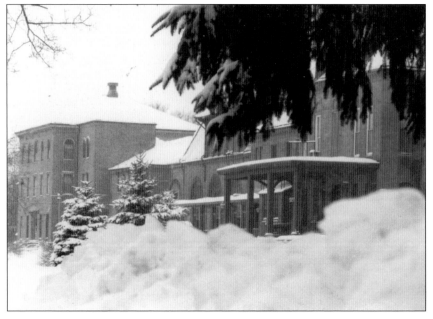

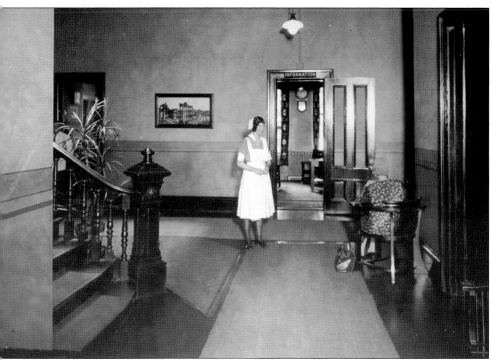

The trustees requested that the state legislature allocate $52.30 per patient (equivalent to $1,402.90 today) in order to purchase beds, bedding, tables, chairs, settees, towels, table linens, crockery and utensils, and toiletry sets for each person. The sheets for the hospital were cut and hemmed at the Reformatory Prison for Women at Sherbourne, a fact of which the trustees were quite proud, having provided meaningful work for another institution. The hospital was lit first by gas fixtures fueled by gasoline that was made on the premises, refined by machine. Speaking tubes were installed that connected the laboratory to all but two of the wards. Those two wards had telephones installed. Ten of the wards had their own fireplaces. (Both, courtesy of Massachusetts Department of Mental Health.)

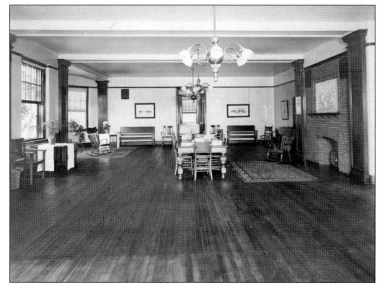

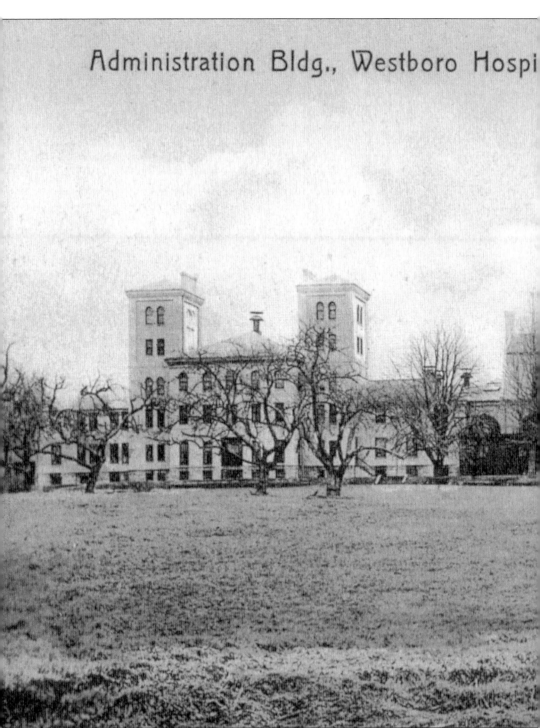

Construction was completed by December 1886, and a reception was held for Gov. George [
Robinson. Even before its opening, the trustees were looking ahead to training physicians i
homeopathy and how best to prevent burnout amongst the attendants, knowing that the patier
numbers would not remain low for long. A few days after the reception, the first 204 patients wei

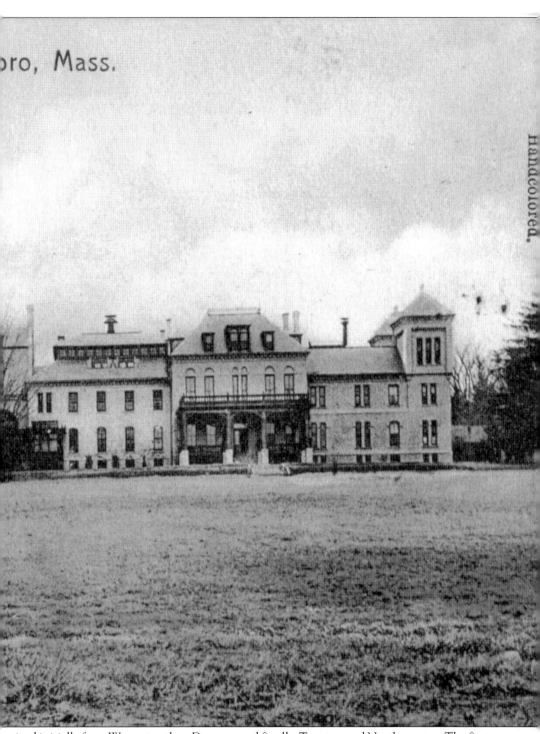

Handcolored.

ceived initially from Worcester, then Danvers, and finally, Taunton and Northampton. The first roup of patients had been deemed "chronic" patients, long-term sufferers of mental illness. In the nd, the hospital was finished at a cost of just $150,000. (Courtesy Westborough Public Library.)

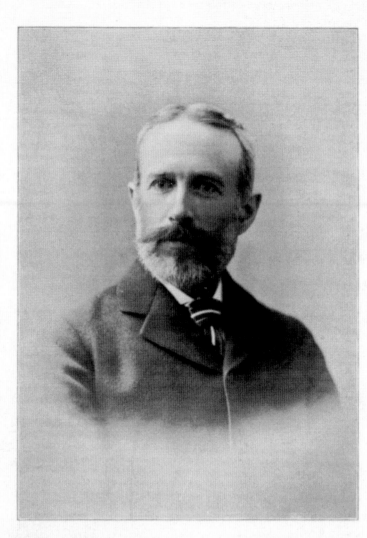

Dr. Nathaniel Emmons Paine was appointed the first superintendent of Westborough. He previously served as the assistant physician at the State Homeopathic Asylum for the Insane in Middletown, New York and accepted the promotion in on May 1, 1886. Ahead of the arrival of patients, Paine requested that the state furnish enough money for a patient library, a carriage for "giving exercise and change of scene to the female and weak patients," a billiards table, an organ for the chapel, and two boats—one for rowing, and one for sailing. Paine immediately set about making connections with local medical schools and hosted clinics in homeopathy as well as took in numerous donations of both money and goods for the hospital. (Courtesy Westborough Public Library.)

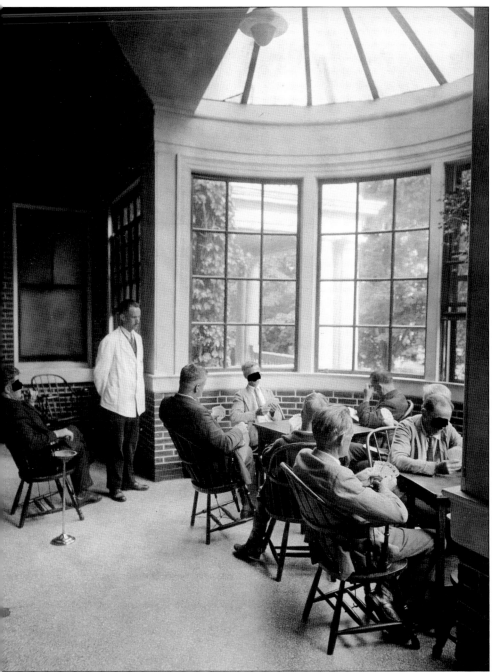

n his capacity as superintendent, Paine made certain that the hospital was equipped to maintain low patient to staff ratio, specifically one hundred patients to every one physician so that the edical staff might devote as much time and attention to individual patients as possible. This also ade the rest cure easier to administer. Each ward had a south-facing day room where patients ould sit for a certain number of hours each day while doctors made their rounds and checked in ith each of them. Paine made certain that every detail on the wards was seen to in meticulous ashion. (Courtesy Massachusetts Department of Mental Health.)

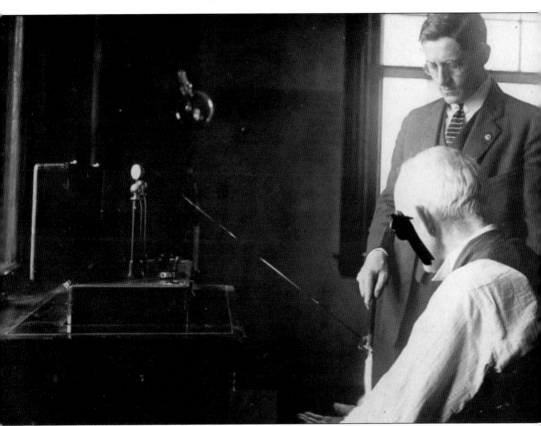

Practitioners of homeopathic medicine generally believed that patients should be treated with only one medicine at a time and that those medicines should be derived from natural substances. Superintendents and medical doctors in the field advocated for "treatment of the insane by mildness rather than coercion," a philosophy that was similar to that of moral treatment, which was the foundation for the many other public asylums that were built on the Kirkbride Plan. However, whereas work and activity were the primary tenets of moral treatment, rest and sleep were paramount in treating insanity at Westborough. (Courtesy Massachusetts Department of Mental Health.)

Two

HOMEOPATHY

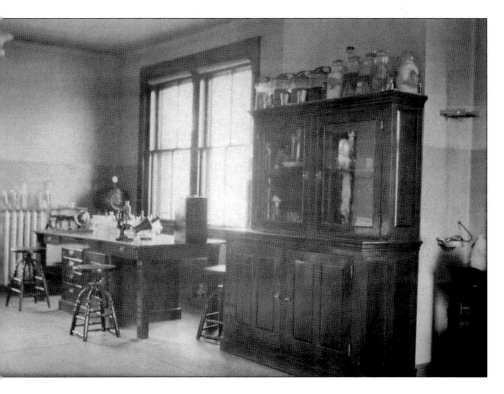

oth homeopathy and the rest cure were incorporated into the treatment model at Westborough.
pon admission, patients were sent to bed and given "milk and good food in abundance." Paine
chewed the use of "hypnotic" sedatives like morphine and opium, as he believed that the forced
iet of these "hypnotics" was not as curative as rest and natural medicines, such as belladonna,
hich was used regularly to treat mania. (Courtesy Massachusetts Department of Mental Health.)

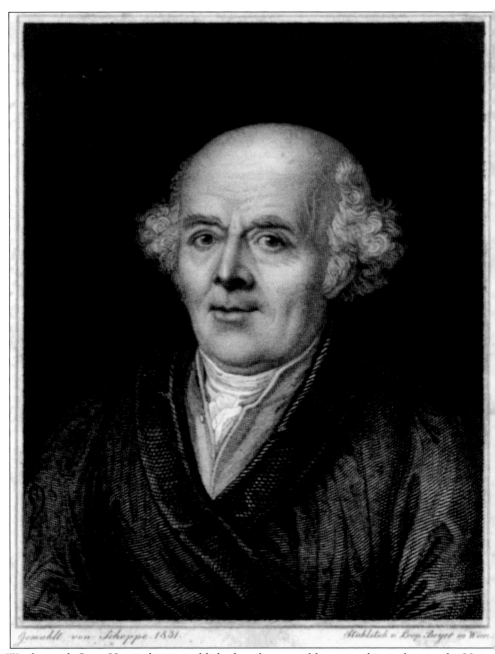

Gemahlt von Schoppe 1831.   Stahlstich v. Leop. Beyer in Wien

Westborough State Hospital was established as the second homeopathic asylum in the United States. Homeopathy was popular in the mid-1800s, introduced by German physician Samuel Hahnemann. Dissatisfied with the medical treatments of his time such as bloodletting, he felt that many of the "modern" treatments often did far more harm than good, and he set out to prove that there were far more rational ways to treat chronic illnesses. Hahnemann accepted a post at an asylum, where he asserted that mental illness was no different from bodily illness, which led him to suggest that mental illness should be cured by physical treatments. Hahnemann is credited as being one of the first to treat the mentally ill humanely; shortly after, Phillippe Pinel unchained the patients at Bicêtre Hospital in France. (Courtesy Wellcome Library.)

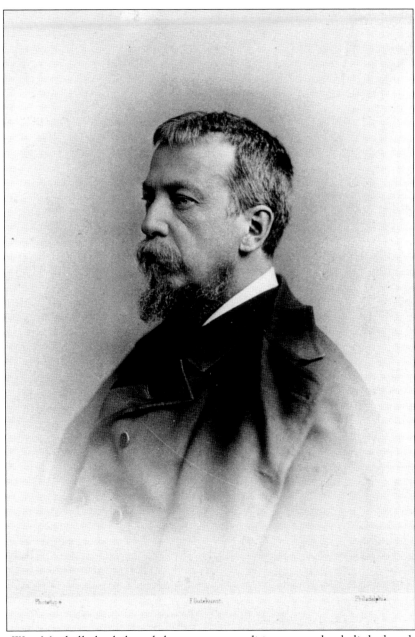

Dr. Silas Weir Mitchell also believed that nervous conditions were closely linked to the health of the physical body. During the Civil War, he was put in charge of "nervous injuries," soldiers who were exhibiting symptoms of mania or delirium. Later, in private practice, he encountered numerous female patients who presented with similar symptoms. Weir Mitchell surmised that if these women were removed from their environments and forced to rest while taking in a hearty diet and being stimulated by both massage and electrotherapy (the use of electrical current to speed the healing of wounds), they would be relieved of the symptoms of hysteria. Weir Mitchell is best known for having treated Charlotte Perkins Gilman, whose own experience with rest cure inspired her most famous short story, *The Yellow Wallpaper*. (Courtesy US National Library of Medicine.)

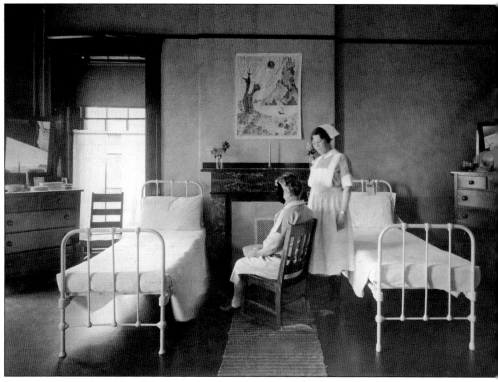

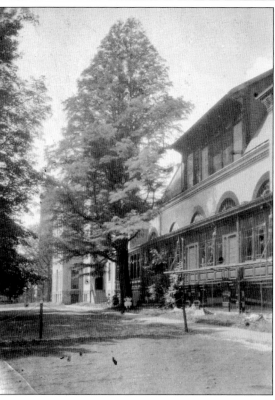

The first annual report notes, "As the cure, in many cases of insanity, depends upon the sleep that is obtained, and as many are easily disturbed in their sleep, this precaution to procure the utmost quiet must be a material advantage." In keeping with this theory, "wickets" (screens) were installed in the doors to aid in nighttime observation without waking the patients. Dr. Paine noted in the hospital's third annual report that "no deviation from true homeopathy has ever been made." Treatment also included massage and electrical stimulation to aid in relaxation. Minute quantities of sleeping medicines were administered to a small number of patients. By and large, the treatment approach was successful, with most patients recovering in three to four months. Within two years, the hospital had discharged a recovered 91 of its more than 400 patients. (Above, courtesy Massachusetts Department of Mental Health; below, courtesy Westborough Public Library.)

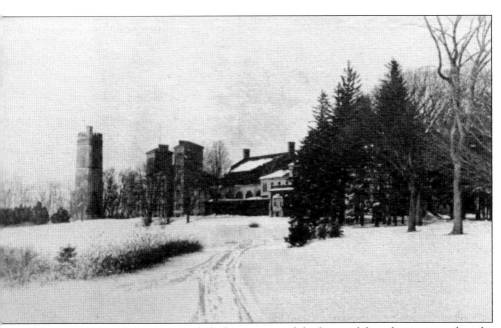

One of Paine's greatest desires was to shift the purpose of the hospital from being an asylum for incurables to a hospital for acute cases. Acute cases were more responsive to homeopathic treatment methods, and Paine suggested that they always be separated from chronic cases, who languished in the asylums. He immediately suggested that a separate building be constructed for chronic cases "on the most distant part of the grounds." (Courtesy Westborough Public Library)

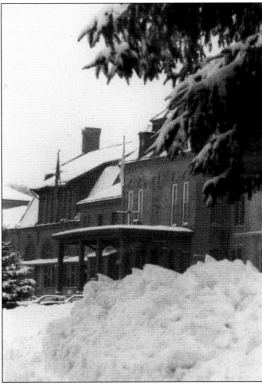

The other of Paine's most pressing suggestions was for the construction of a separate asylum for "inebriates," or alcoholics. In spite of their struggles with their addiction, Paine believed them to be largely of sound mind and unjustly detained in a hospital for the insane. He further believed that alcoholics required specialized treatment to overcome their addiction that could not be provided by the insane hospital. (Courtesy Massachusetts Department of Mental Health.)

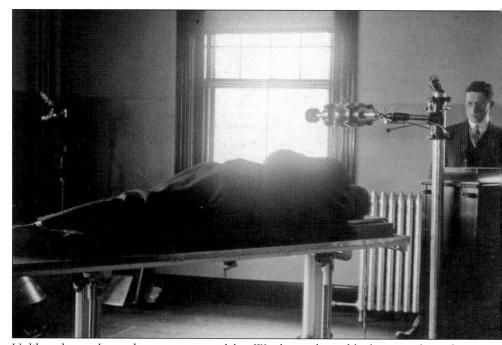

Unlike other asylums, the treatment model at Westborough used little to no physical restraint. Restraint might only be used if a patient on rest cure became restless or violent. Then they might be wrapped in a bed sheet until they were calm. As well, if a patient were to engage regularly in "bad practices," such as masturbation, they might be placed in canvas undergarments to discourage the behavior. (Courtesy Massachusetts Department of Mental Health)

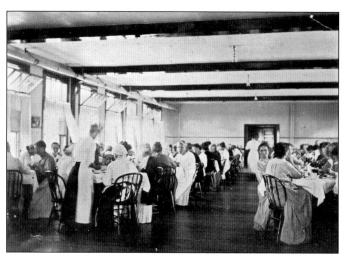

Another unique feature at Westborough was the use of the congregate model for meals. More than 200 patients, both male and female, took their meals in the large dining hall that was attached to the main kitchen. In other hospitals, patients remained segregated on the wards for meals, which were transported to them from the main kitchen. (Courtesy Westborough Public Library.)

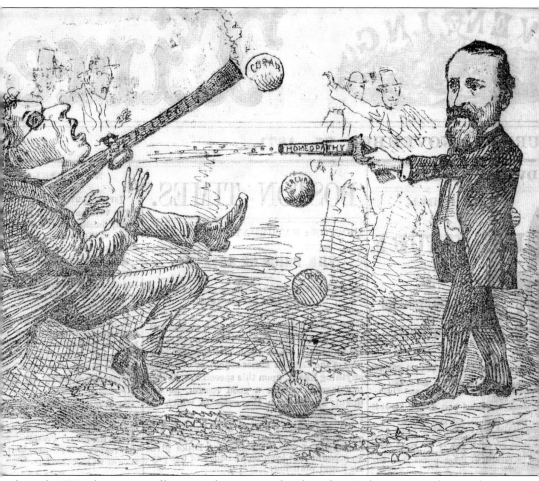

In the early 1870s, the practice of homeopathy was considered conduct "unbecoming and unworthy of an honorable physician," and the Massachusetts Medical Society sought to have practitioners banned from the group, including I.T. Talbot, who would later play a large part in the history of Westborough. However, by April 1887, amidst the controversy surrounding homeopathy, Westborough hosted a meeting of the State Homeopathic Medical Society, which attracted more than 200 attendees. Paine wanted other homeopathic physicians to have the chance to see the wards and learn about the treatment programs at the hospital; the event was deemed a success, and Paine noted in the annual report that "It was enjoyed by none more than by the patients." (Courtesy Massachusetts Homeopathic Medical Society.)

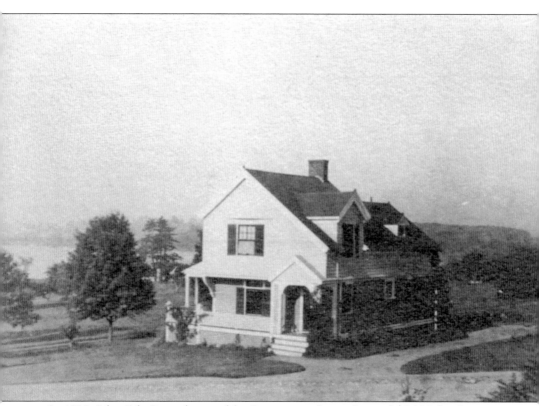

In 1890, John Felt Osgood, a wealthy Boston merchant, donated $3,000 for the construction of a private cottage overlooking the lake for patients who needed "quiet isolation and careful attendance." An architect's rendering and floor plan were included in the annual report of 1891 as construction was underway. Its design was quintessential Queen Anne with an asymmetrical roofline dressed in both clapboards and shingles. The cottage was completed by the next year and occupied by a single patient, an attendant, and a cook. Designed by Stephen Earle of Worcester, it contained a first-floor parlor and kitchen with three bedrooms on the second floor. (Courtesy Westborough Public Library.)

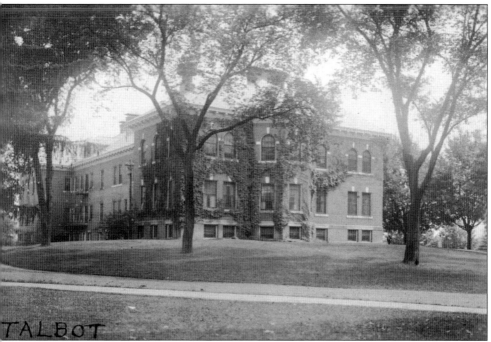

TALBOT

Hydrotherapy played a large part in the treatment at Westborough. In 1896, the trustees requested funds to erect a building for the acutely insane at a cost of $50,000. The building would be fitted with Turkish bathrooms as well as spray baths. Continuous flow baths were used frequently to bring down body temperatures when patients were agitated. The building was completed in March 1898 and named for Dr. Israel Tisdale Talbot. In April 1899, the *New England Medical Gazette* praised the Talbot Building, saying it should be noted that it is "a State building, built with public money, and has been entirely finished within the original appropriations." It was the first building in the state for the segregation of recent cases from others. (Both, courtesy Westborough Public Library.)

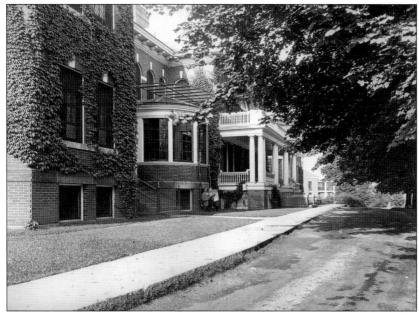

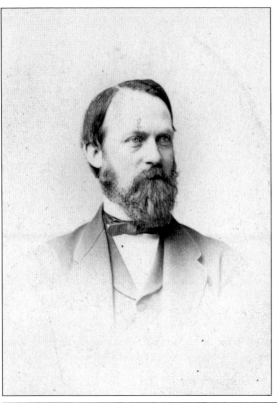

In order to provide the broadest scope of treatment, the hospital administration formed a consulting board of physicians and surgeons in an "attempt to place [Westborough] in professional relations with men engaged in the active practice of medicine and surgery." The board was chaired by Dr. Israel Tisdale Talbot, whose wife, Emily, served on the board of trustees. Dr. Talbot not only chaired the consulting board but was also instrumental in securing the initial legislation necessary to establish Westborough. His sudden death in 1898 was marked as a great loss to the entire state hospital, and he was memorialized in the annual report of 1899 by both the trustees and the superintendent. (Above, courtesy of Countway Library of Medicine; below, courtesy Massachusetts Department of Mental Health.)

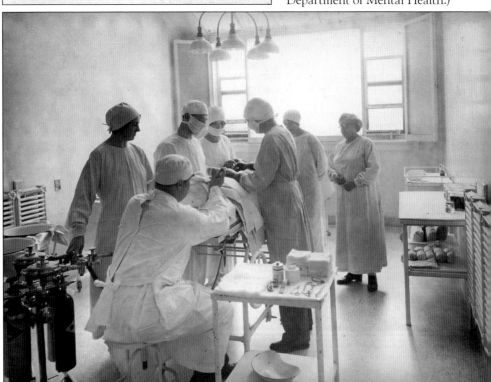

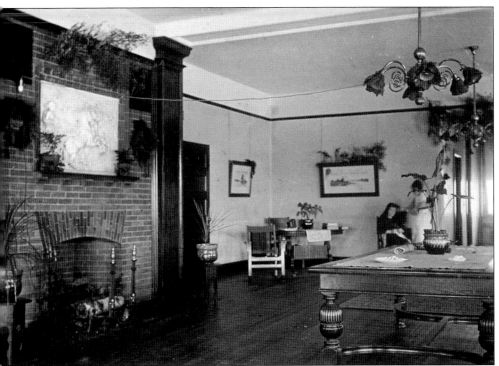

The common areas of Talbot Building were richly appointed and furnished nearly identically in both the east and west wings. Each common area had a fireplace and billiards table as well as a sitting area for reading or writing letters. A furniture shop was also established in the basement of the Talbot Building, which was formerly occupied by the occupational therapy department. The occupational therapy department was moved to a larger space in the main administration building. Volleyball equipment was also purchased and installed on the front lawn of Talbot, and patients with grounds privileges were allowed access to the tennis courts. (Both, courtesy Massachusetts Department of Mental Health.)

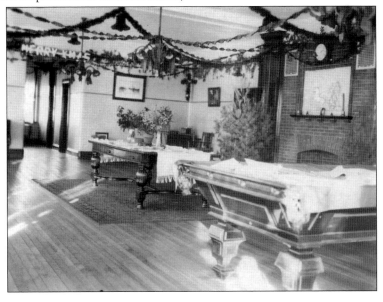

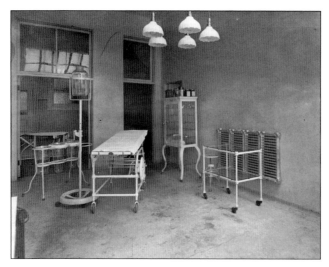

Once the hospital was fully electrified, static and high-frequency electrical waves were used in the treatment of many patients who were diagnosed with minor depression and/or insomnia. The electricity was used to stimulate healing within the body and was often coupled with massage. Eventually, the hospital purchased electric massaging machines to make the treatment more readily accessible to a greater number of patients. (Courtesy Massachusetts Department of Mental Health.)

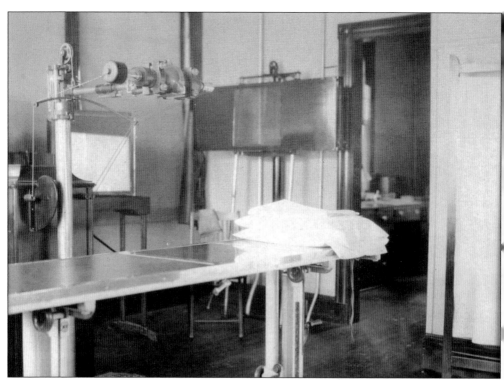

In the early 1930s, the medical staff began experimenting with fever therapies and colonic irrigation. Fever is considered the body's oldest and most primitive mechanism for fighting infection, and doctors believed that by inducing a fever, the body might heal itself of psychotic symptoms. The therapies were short-lived, and the hospital returned to a strict homeopathic basis for treatment. (Courtesy Massachusetts Department of Mental Health.)

In the early 1900s, the hospital began using a new system of classifying mental illnesses established by German psychiatrist Emil Kraeplin, who was credited with labeling two distinct forms of insanity: manic depression and dementia praecox. Dementia Praecox was the predominant diagnosis for many years and was applied broadly to patients displaying a number of different symptoms. It was eventually reclassified as schizophrenia, and the symptoms more specifically defined. Dr. Solomon Carter Fuller, who later served as the hospital's pathologist, would take a sabbatical in 1905 in order to study with Kraeplin. Fuller was best known for his groundbreaking research into the disease now known as Alzheimer's. (Both, courtesy John Gray.)

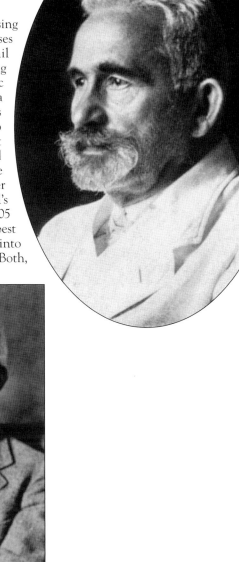

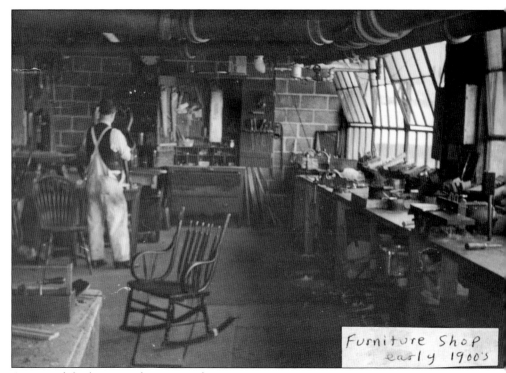

Furniture Shop early 1900's

As part of the homeopathic approach to treatment, patients were assigned occupational work, which was considered essential to a patient's recovery. The hospital included a shoe shop, a furniture shop (pictured above), and a sewing room. Patients worked in the gardens and did all the mending and sewing on campus. They also wove rugs, did leather work, and made arts and crafts. Later, a mattress shop would be added as well as a space to manufacture brooms and brushes. In the furniture shop, patients repaired furniture including caning and upholstery. Dr. Paine remarked in 1905 that "employment is the best medicine for the chronic insane." Much like subscribers of moral treatment and the Kirkbride Plan, Paine believed that it promoted quiet and lessened the intensity of delusions. (Above, courtesy of Massachusetts Department of Mental Health; below, courtesy of Phil Kittredge.)

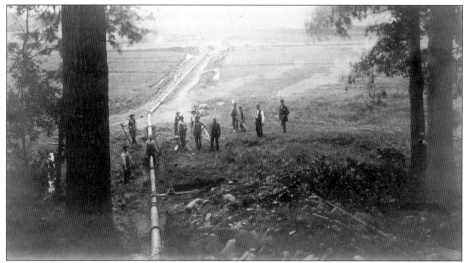

Three

THE HOSPITAL
ON THE LAKE

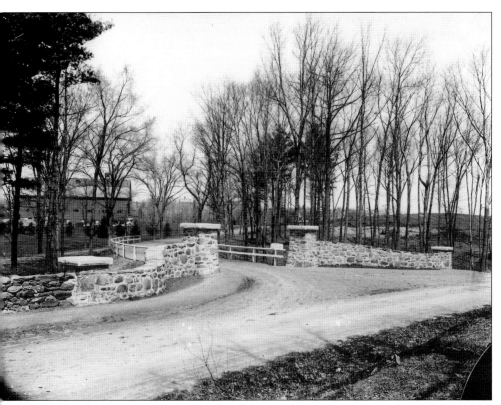

The Westborough Insane Hospital was officially opened in a ceremony on December 1, 1886, which was presided over by then governor George D. Robinson. The first patients received were transferred from Worcester State Hospital on December 6, and by the end of the fiscal year, there were 313 patients at Westborough. (Courtesy Phil Kittredge.)

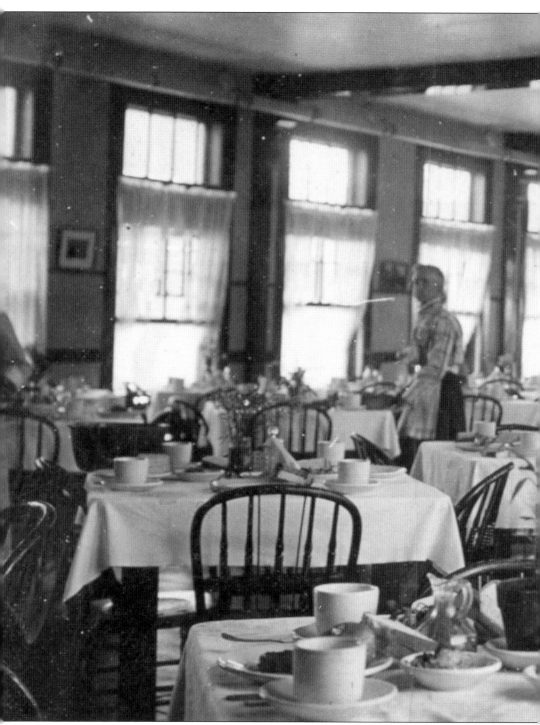

The newly formed Westborough Insane Hospital filled rapidly and was deemed overcrowded by the close of its third year of operation. The population peaked at 507 patients on September 26 1888, and did not decrease again. The most crowded were the wards for the violent, noisy, and "demented" patients. A statistical table provided in the annual reports of the time listed the

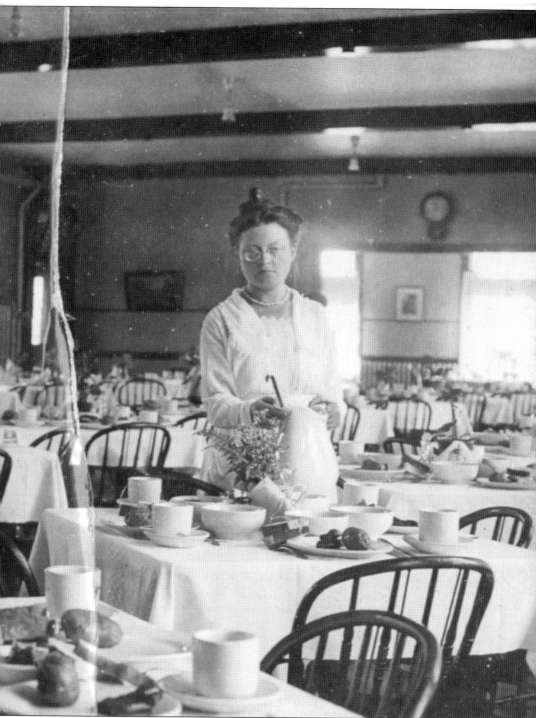

following as reasons for commitment: business trouble (4 men, 1 woman), disappointment in love (2 women), masturbation (14 men, 8 women), and overstudy (3 women). Dr. Paine began suggesting that the "propagation of the insane" be limited, as too many children born to insane women were themselves later deemed insane. (Courtesy Massachusetts Department of Mental Health.)

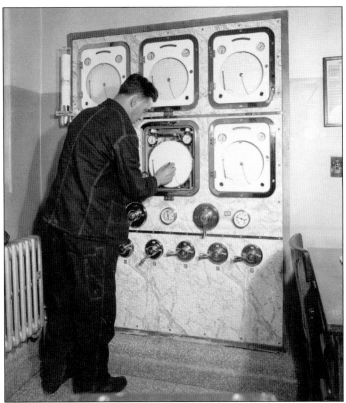

Despite the overcrowding, treatment continued without the use of hypnotic drugs and without increased use of restraint. Some patients were successfully boarded out to local families in order to make space on the wards, and one-third of those who remained were gainfully employed on the wards as well as in the kitchen, dining room, and laundry pictured here. (Courtesy Massachusetts Department of Mental Health.)

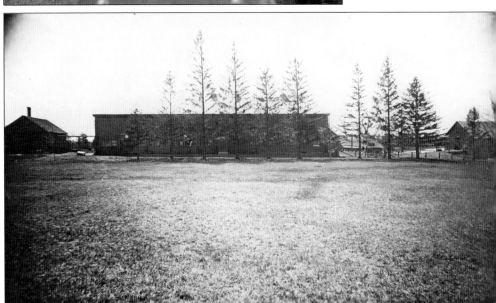

The overcrowding affected the staff as well as the patients, creating less than favorable living circumstances for not only the nurses but also the medical staff. Dr. Paine and his family were living in two rooms that adjoined a parlor and dining room while the assistant physician, George Adams, lived in one room while his wife and child lived in part of one of the cottages on the property. (Courtesy Phil Kittredge.)

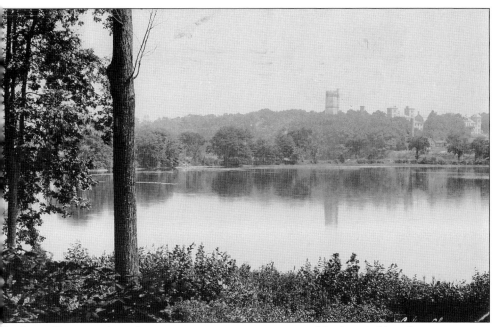

The first addition made to the campus was not an expansion of the hospital but the construction of a 70-foot water tower, which was painted yellow to match the hospital. The hospital would struggle for years to find an adequate water supply that would provide water clean enough to drink and bathe in while also supplying the volume needed to power the steam heat and do the washing up. (Courtesy Phil Kittredge.)

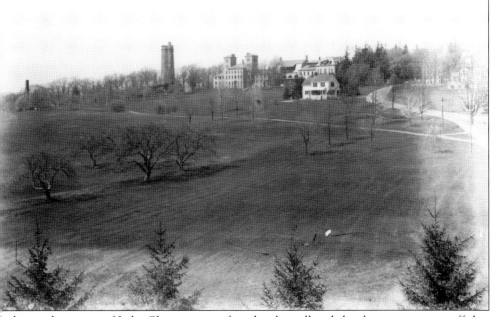

Early on, the waters of Lake Chauncy were found to be polluted thanks to sewage runoff that was being deposited in the lake. It was presumed that this pollution was directly responsible for an outbreak of typhoid fever in 1901. The lake was officially condemned by the State Board of Health as an unfit water source in 1905. (Courtesy Phil Kittredge.)

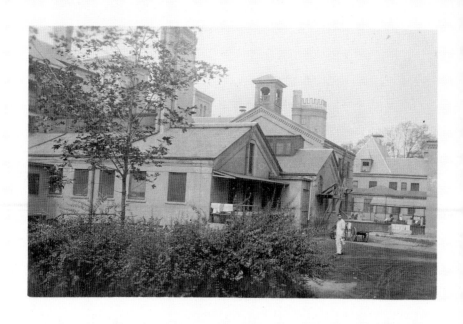

When the reform school kitchen was cleared away, the hospital set about building a new kitchen complete with bakery and food storage. The above image was taken as the construction of the kitchen was in progress. It was built immediately to the rear of the first-floor congregate dining hall and connected to the main building by above-ground corridors. The original laundry was on the first floor of the rear center beneath the ward for working male patients. The laundry was divided into washing, drying, and ironing rooms. The drying of the linens was achieved by using the heat from steam pipes that ran throughout the laundry. (Both, courtesy Massachusetts Department of Mental Health.)

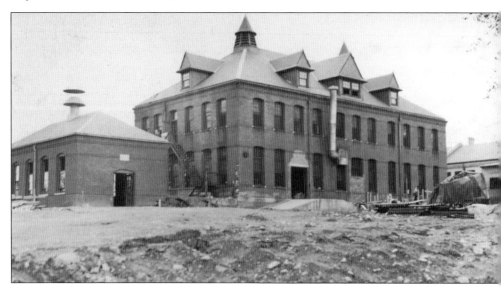

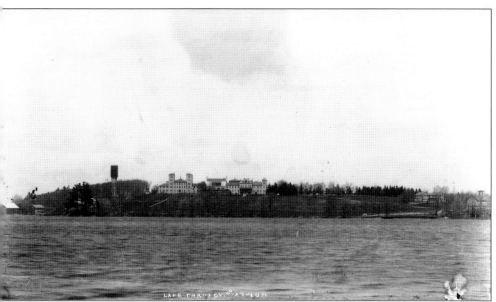

Much of the overcrowding on the wards was relieved by bringing the patients outside as much as possible, both for work and for recreation. A private beach on Lake Chauncy gave patients the opportunity to go boating and swimming. Attendants also frequently took patients out for picnics and baseball games. Dr. Adams suggested a greenhouse be added to the grounds as well. (Courtesy Phil Kittredge.)

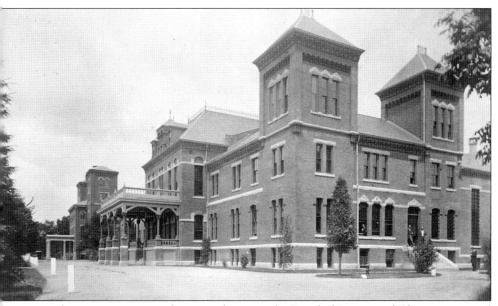

Despite regular successes presented in annual reports, the Board of Lunacy and Charity countered with a number of concerns; chief of which was the "excessive use of restraint and violence." The trustees believed the board's criticisms stemmed from a lack of understanding of homeopathic treatment. The trustees reminded the board that the rest cure required regular restraint and isolation. They also reminded the board of their impressive discharge rate. (Courtesy Phil Kittredge.)

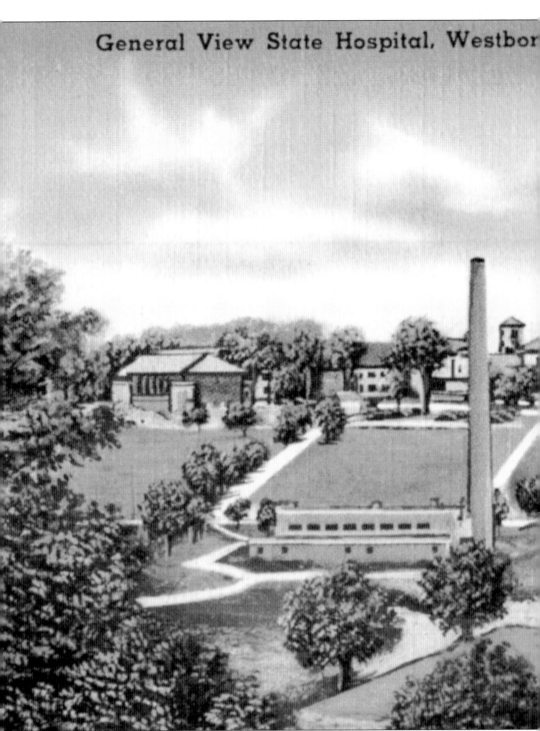

The Board of Lunacy and Charity was also displeased with the level of "noise and confusion" or the wards. The trustees reminded them that they did not use hypnotics and that it was far bette to submit to noise and "apparent confusion" than to risk curability by using medications. The eschewed the use of medications to exercise control over the patients. The trustees also felt pressec

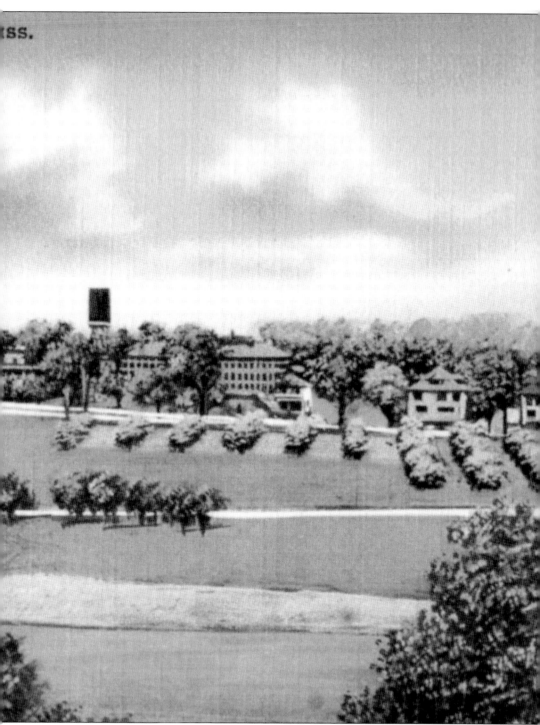

to defend the hospital when the board made mention of the overcrowding as well as the overall cleanliness of the wards. The trustees reminded the board that they were the only hospital that had not been given a new building, nor had their requests for hospital expansion been granted. (Courtesy Westborough Public Library.)

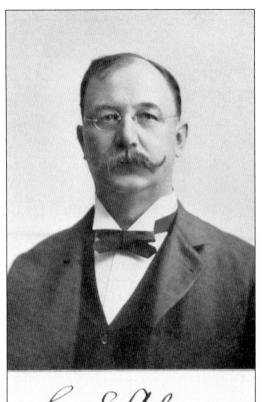

After just five years as superintendent, Dr. Nathaniel Emmons Paine resigned from Westborough State Hospital in 1892. Dr. George S. Adams was promoted to superintendent in time to graduate the first class of nurses from the newly established training program. Paine went on to establish the Newton Nervine, a private hospital for the care of nervous cases. He also became the chairman of the board of trustees of Westborough Insane Hospital. In 1926, Paine was invited to give a presentation for the hospital's 40th anniversary, in which he reviewed his years as superintendent as well as his time serving on the board of trustees. (Left, courtesy Westborough Public Library; below, courtesy Katherine Anderson.)

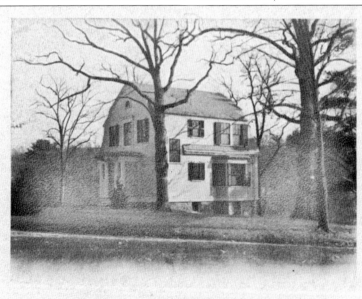

NEWTON NERVINE. NEW COTTAGE FOR ONE PATIENT.
DR. N. EMMONS PAINE.   WEST NEWTON, MASS. (NEAR BOSTON.)

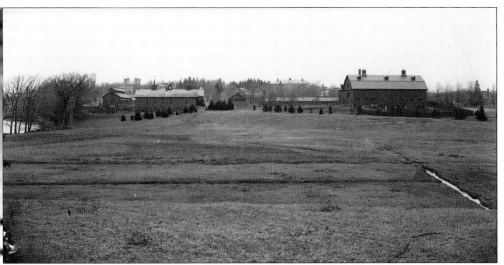

In 1891, just a year before Paine's departure, the board of trustees recommended the purchase of a nearby family farm. The hospital acquired the Stanley House and farm for $8,000. The land was absorbed into the existing farm, and the Stanley House was used as a dorm for "quiet patients." (Courtesy Phil Kittredge.)

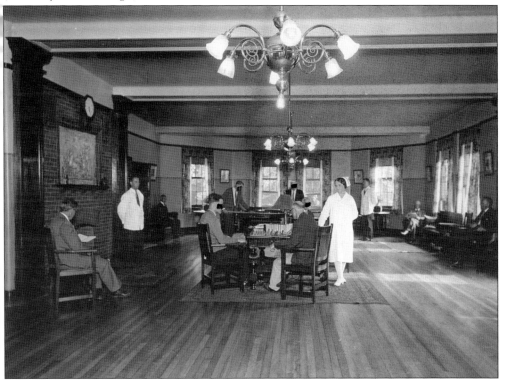

The 10th annual report, released in 1894, was a landmark report, as the trustees were able to announce that, for the first time, Westborough Insane Hospital was in the black. Rather than running at a constant deficit, the hospital had turned a small profit, and with an additional appropriation from the legislature, the gas lighting was updated to electricity. The hospital was fully electrified by October 1894. (Courtesy Massachusetts Department of Mental Health.)

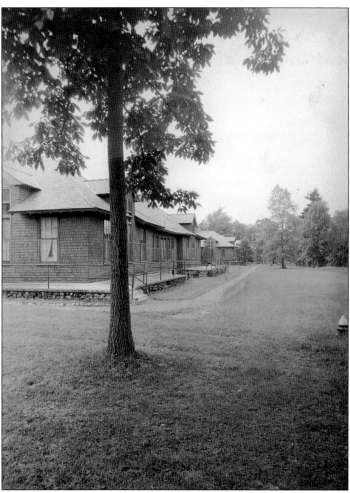

In the early 1900s, Westborough State Hospital was ready to expand its footprint, as well as its farming operations, by purchasing a tract of farmland on the opposite shore of Lake Chauncy. The trustees acquired the Warren and Hollis Farms in 1901. Renovations on the Speare and Dewson Buildings were completed by 1902, followed by construction of the Richmond Colony for women in 1903. Richmond consisted of four cottages for 25 women, each connected to one another by corridors. Both the Warren and Richmond Colonies were occupied by "quiet cases," who required little supervision and were able to work. (Courtesy Massachusetts Department of Mental Health.)

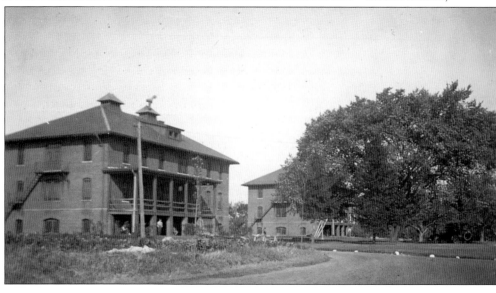

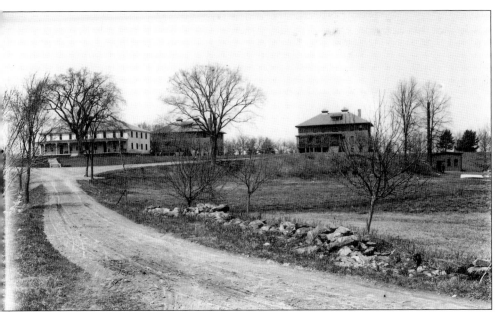

The Warren Colony, consisting of the original Warren farmhouse and the Speare and Dewson Cottages, was complete in 1902. After acquiring the land, the farmhouse was enlarged and completely remodeled in order to accommodate 35 male patients. Two more cottages (Speare and Dewson) were then designed by Kendall, Taylor, and Stevens to house another 100 men of the "chronic working class." The home-like cottages were completely open and afforded the patients a great deal of freedom and privilege. A small tuberculosis sanitarium for men was also attached to the Warren Colony. Each of the detached colonies had its own kitchen and dining halls as well as their own sewage disposal systems. (Above, courtesy Phil Kittredge; below courtesy Massachusetts Department of Mental Health.)

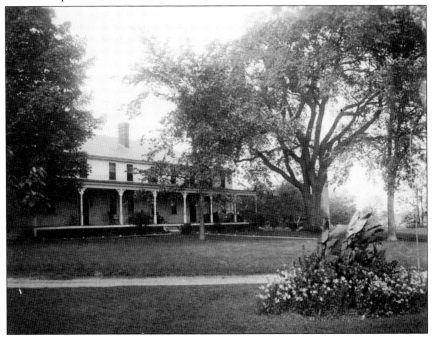

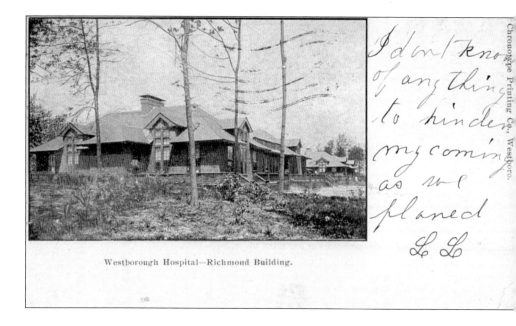

I don't know of anything to hinder my coming as we planed L L

Westborough Hospital—Richmond Building.

Once the Warren Colony was proven a success, the land for the Richmond Colony on the opposite shore of Lake Chauncy was purchased for $3,000 and named for former trustee George B. Richmond. The four cottages were erected along with a sanitarium for 20 women with tuberculosis. A laundry facility was also added in order to relieve some of the workload in the main laundry. The Richmond Colony also housed the shoe shop where all patient and employee shoes were repaired and cleaned. Basket making was also quickly introduced with the hope that it would occupy a great deal of the occupational work at the Richmond Colony. (Above, courtesy Westborough Public Library; below, courtesy Phil Kittredge.)

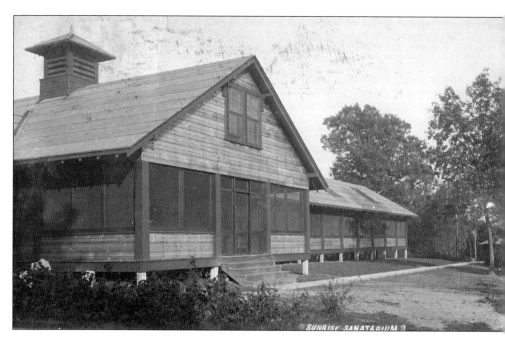

SUNRISE SANATARIUM

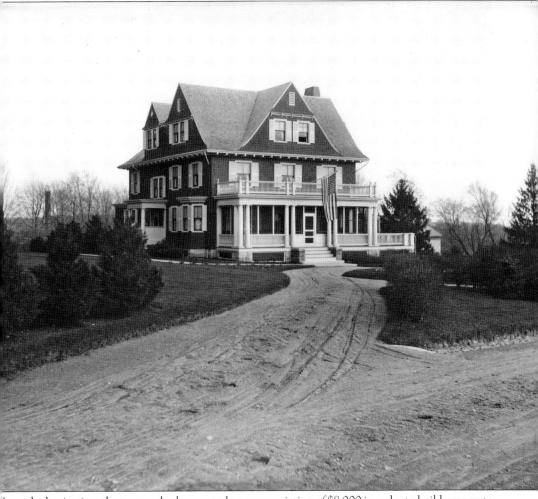

From the beginning, the trustees had requested an appropriation of $8,000 in order to build a separate cottage for the superintendent. By now, George S. Adams had been serving as superintendent since Dr. Paine's resignation in 1892. Adams took a brief leave of absence after contracting typhoid fever in 1902 but returned to his post a year later when the trustees renewed their request for a superintendent's home. In their request, the trustees noted that after 17 years of service, "It is due him and his family that a suitable home should be provided outside of the walls of the administration building." (Courtesy Phil Kittredge.)

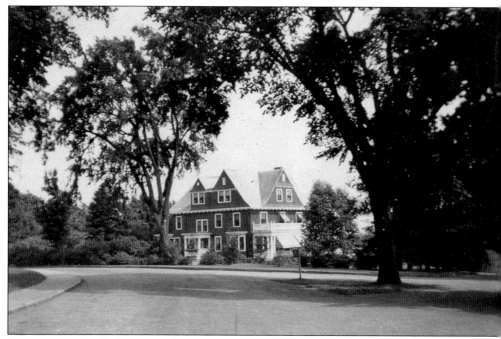

Construction finally began on the superintendent's cottage in 1904 and was finished by spring of the next year. Dr. Adams and his family moved into a fully furnished home; however, it was noted a short time later that, in spite of the comfortable accommodations, the superintendent was making $500 per year less than superintendents of hospitals in other states on the East Coast. (Courtesy Westborough Public Library.)

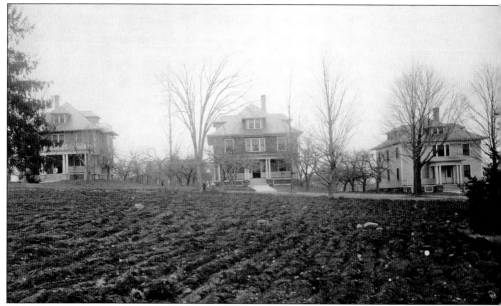

As the campus grew, so did the attendant workforce who were, up until the early 1900s, living side by side on the wards with the patients. By 1904, the first three nurses' homes were constructed, providing quarters for 54 nurses. Much of the work was performed by patients under the supervision of the hospital's maintenance department. (Courtesy Massachusetts Department of Mental Health.)

56

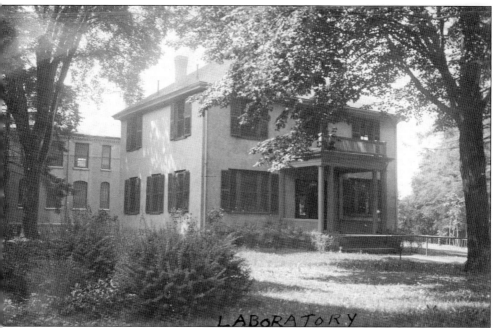

LABORATORY

In 1902, funds were appropriated to construct "better accommodations" for the pathologist as well as an updated operating room to be built on the foundation of the Peters House directly across the way from the Talbot and Codman Buildings. The pathologist was working under less than desirable conditions in the main administration building, and as research was becoming a major focus at Westborough, it was deemed necessary to have a larger, more modern space for conducting that research. The pathology lab regularly performed tests of the blood and urine, as well as a large number of autopsies. The lab would also eventually house the pharmacy where the natural cures used in the hospital were bottled and stored. (Above, courtesy Westborough Public Library; below, courtesy Massachusetts Department of Mental Health.)

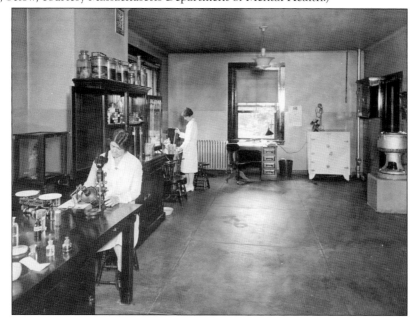

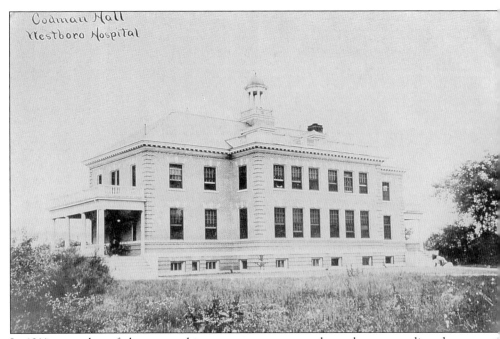

Codman Hall
Westboro Hospital

In 1911, a number of changes and improvements were made, such as expanding the women wards to accommodate the nearly 1,200 patients. A porch was also added to Codman (above as seen in the image below. In August 1911, the hospital suffered a blow when a new law wa enacted governing the use of restraint. While it reduced the number of restraints, the number c patient to patient assaults and injuries to staff increased in kind. Supt. George Adams believe that in acute cases when all else failed restraint was ultimately the only humane solution, but h was willing to abolish restraints in chronic cases. (Above, courtesy Westborough Public Library below, courtesy Phil Kittredge.)

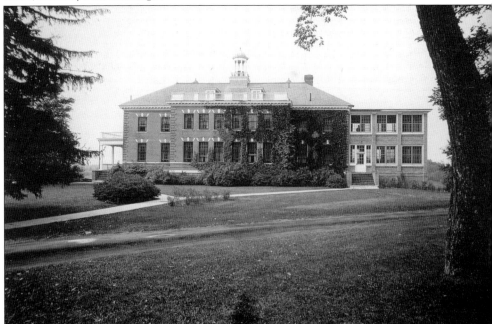

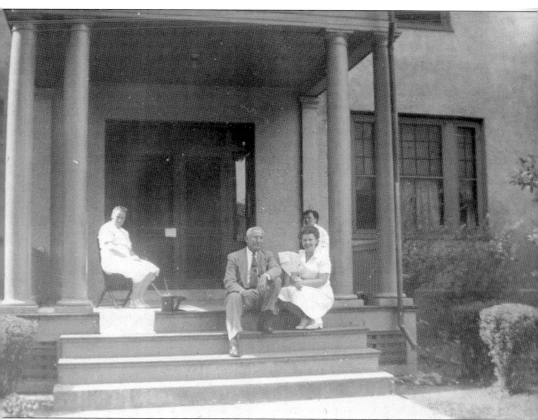

n February 1, 1921, Dr. Lydia B. Pierce was appointed pathologist after the position had remained
en for many months. Prior to her arrival, the lab was completely renovated, and the equipment
as updated. In 1924, Dr. Pierce presented a paper at the spring meeting of the Massachusetts
omoeopathic Medical Society on "unusual material" found during the autopsy of a patient
ith Hodgkin's disease. Dr. Pierce presented a second unusual case at a meeting of the American
ychiatric Association in Atlantic City in June of that same year. The second paper was then
blished in the *American Journal of Psychiatry*. Dr. Pierce served as pathologist for 32 years and
tired in 1953. (Courtesy Westborough Public Library.)

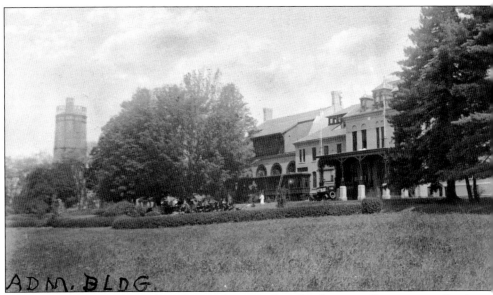

ADM. BLDG.

The superintendent was not the only one who was affected by low overall wages rates. On August 1, 1906, the legislature passed a law that employees could not work longer than an eight-hour workday, which meant the hospital would have to hire more attendants to cover the newly formed schedules. However, the salaries were still comparatively low, and the hospital struggled to attract quality attendants as they had "by no means kept pace with the general increase of wages." It was equally difficult for the hospital to attract married couples, as there was no housing available for couples. If married employees wished to take advantage of the room and board included in their wages, they would have to live separately on the wards. The first cottage for married couples was constructed in 1909. (Above, courtesy Westborough Public Library; below, courtesy Massachusetts Department of Mental Health.)

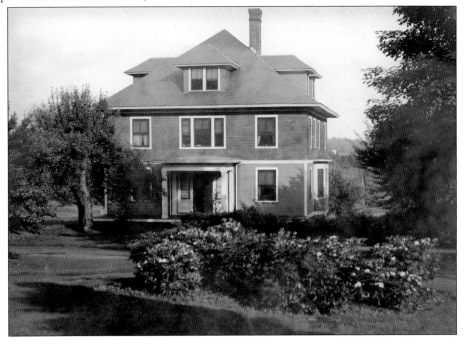

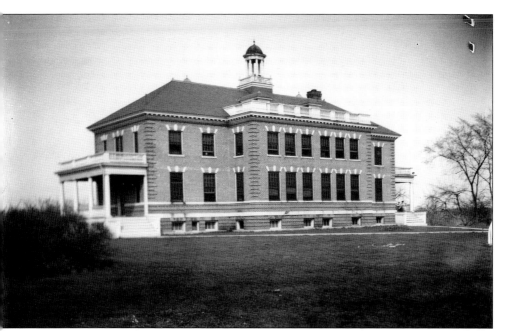

Pleased with the success of the Talbot Building for acute cases, the trustees suggested that a similar building for acute disturbed cases be built behind Talbot, similar in structure but made of concrete and cement inside. The building was finished and occupied by the next year, and it was named for the Honorable Charles R. Codman, a former trustee who was now a member of the State Board of Insanity. (Courtesy Phil Kittredge.)

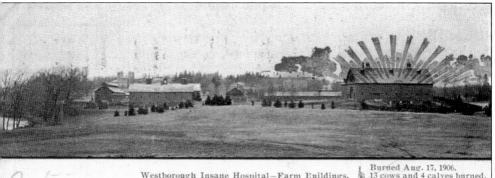

Westborough Insane Hospital—Farm Buildings.

Burned Aug. 17, 1906.
13 cows and 4 calves burned.
Loss about $14,000.

Chronotype Printing Co., Westboro.

One of the chief concerns noted in multiple annual reports was fire safety. On August 17, 1906, a fire ripped through the cattle barn destroying it completely, killing "seventeen head of stock" and destroying a good deal of grain and hay. The monetary loss to the hospital was estimated to be $14,000. The next recorded fire was on November 13, 1914, which resulted in the death of a hospital employee. (Courtesy John Gray.)

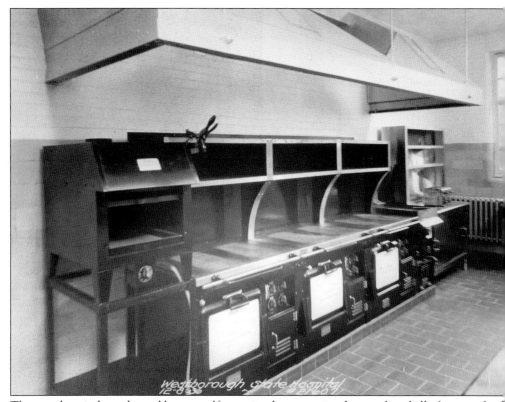

The state hospital was, by and large, a self-contained community that produced all of its own food on site. The hospital had its own in-house bakery that produced all the hospital's bread. Initially, the bakery was housed in the same building as the laundry, both of which were updated first in 1893. In 1907, the trustees requested $6,500 to build and equip a new, much larger bakery. While it was being constructed, a portable oven was used. When completed, the bakery also housed the laundry and boiler house. A new kitchen was also constructed with a larger cafeteria attached to accommodate the growing hospital population. (Both, courtesy Massachusetts Department of Mental Health.)

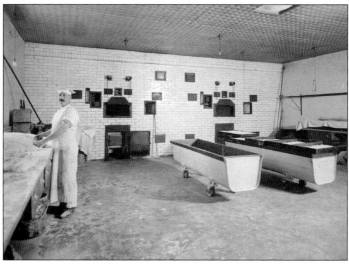

By 1908, nearly every building on the hospital campus was overcrowded. Talbot was full, and Osgood Cottage was pressed into service as housing for six patients as opposed to one. Codman was also full, and the hospital was in need of a similar building for "disturbed" male patients. The women's wards in the main hospital building were also overcrowded, and the old wards were in desperate need of refurbishing. (Courtesy Massachusetts Department of Mental Health.)

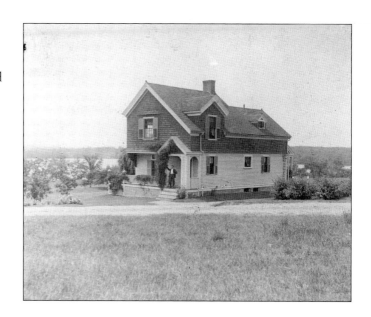

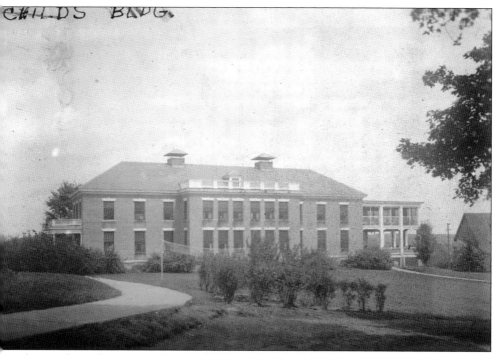

In order to relieve the overcrowding in Codman, the Childs Building was constructed, and the acute female cases were moved to the new building, leaving Codman to become the new home for acute male cases. Childs was a "thoroughly up-to-date" two-story hospital building with grill enclosed veranda, provisions for hydrotherapy, and an electrotherapy suite. (Courtesy Westborough Public Library.)

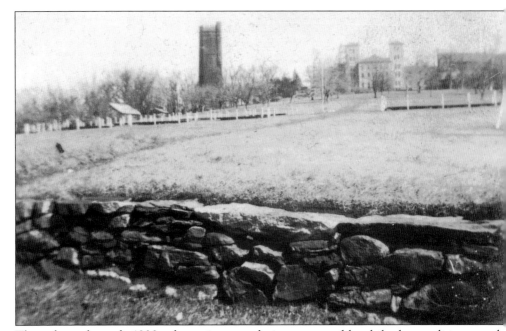

Throughout the early 1900s, the patient population rose steadily while the conditions on th wards were regularly described as "intolerable," especially the women's wards. In spite of this, th legislature continually changed the laws concerning commitment and continually transferre different classes of patients to Westborough, including alcoholics and "narcotic habitués." (Courtes Westborough Public Library.)

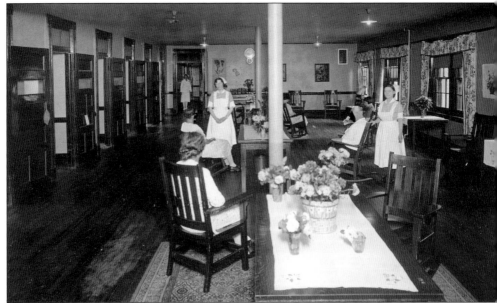

The State Board of Lunacy and Charity, in speaking of the Westborough Insane Hospital in on of its annual reports, made the assertion that "in some of the essential features of a good hospita this institution is sadly lacking." The trustees were certain that the board was alone in tha opinion, though the sentiment was felt, as the board repeatedly denied requests for appropriation (Courtesy Massachusetts Department of Mental Health.)

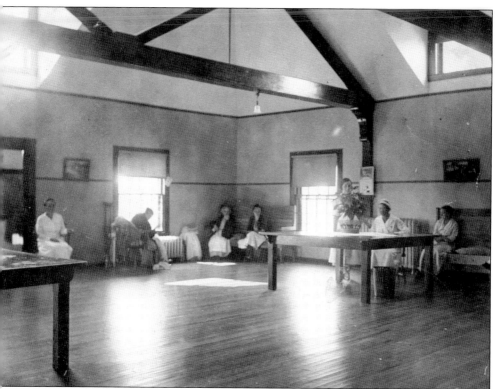

The trustees frequently requested increased appropriations in order to expand the hospital. They bluntly reminded the State Board of Lunacy and Charity that being tight with appropriations would lead to greater expense later. The state continued to refuse appropriations while the trustees' responsibilities increased, forcing some of them to resign. The overcrowding still did not change the mission of the hospital and patients continued to enjoy time outdoors, relatively low staff to patient ratios, and no deviation from the tenets of homeopathic treatment. Many of the patients and their families took the time to thank the staff on leaving the hospital; some even made donations as did their family and friends. (Both, courtesy Massachusetts Department of Mental Health.)

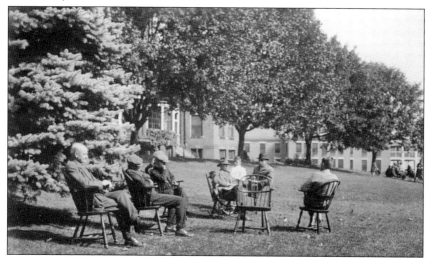

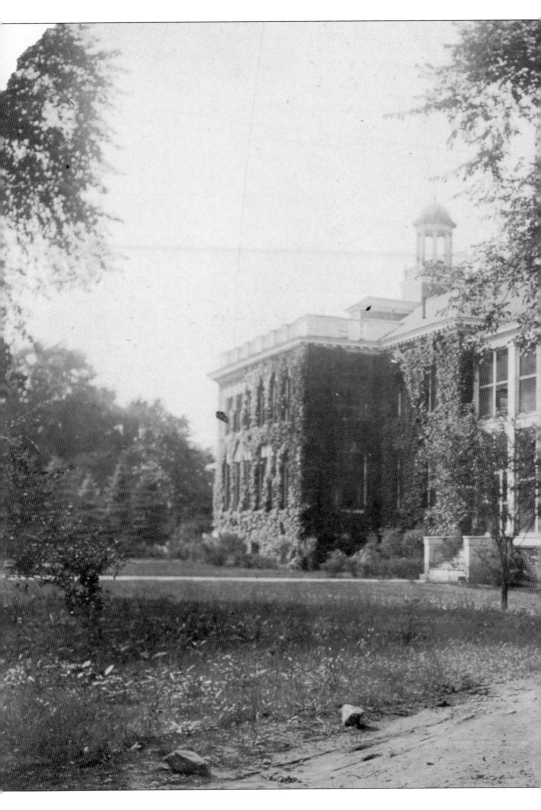

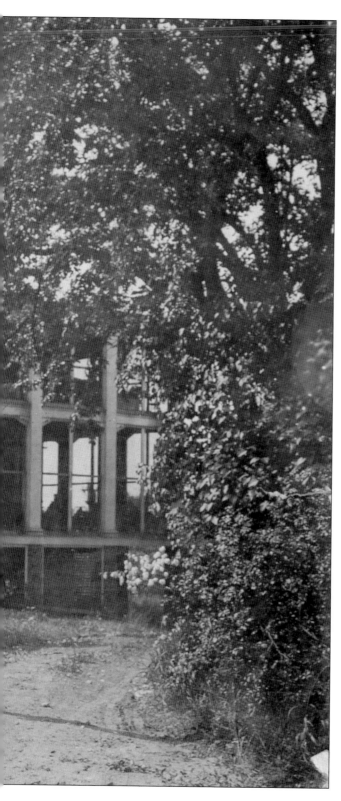

Despite these near constant increases in population as well as continued wage disparities, the hospital still did not deviate from homeopathic treatment. A large percentage of patients worked out of doors, a treatment second only to hydrotherapy, and 11 of the now 49 wards were open (unlocked) wards. Nearly 300 patients had grounds privileges, and during the summer and fall months, 70 male patients were allowed to "camp out" on the old ball grounds on the banks of Lake Chauncy. Patients continued to work both on the farm in the patient gardens while also taking rides into town and at times even out to Worcester. (Courtesy Westborough Public Library.)

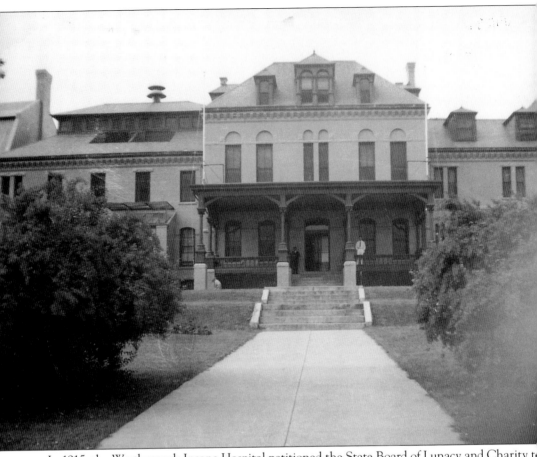

In 1915, the Westborough Insane Hospital petitioned the State Board of Lunacy and Charity to change the hospital's name. Westborough State Hospital, as it was now called, celebrated its 30th anniversary on December 7, 1916, by welcoming a number of visitors who attended presentations by the medical staff. World War I was in full swing and the hospital collected money for yarn and materials to make garments and send supplies to the Red Cross. A number of staff members enlisted in the armed forces, and a substantially depleted workforce was left to care for the nearly 2,000 patients on the wards. (Courtesy Mike Minicucci.)

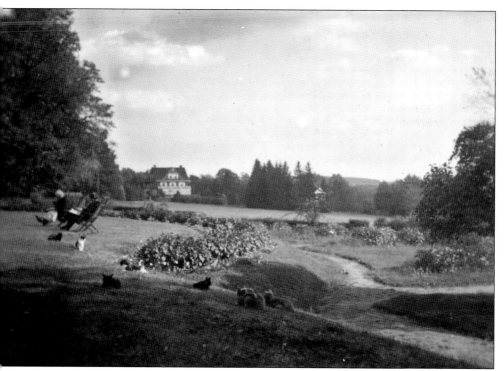

After the war, Dr. Walter Lang replaced Dr. Harry Spalding as superintendent of Westborough after his discharge from the Army. He had previously served as assistant physician at the Homeopathic State Hospital for the Insane in Allentown, Pennsylvania, and the trustees believed him to be unusually well prepared for his post. He is seen here out on the lawns of the superintendent's house. (Courtesy Massachusetts Department of Mental Health.)

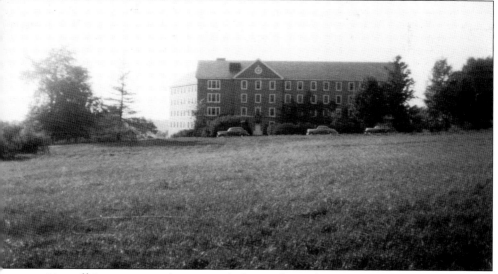

In recognition of his many years of service to the hospital as its first superintendent, then chairman of the board of trustees, and a member of the consulting board of physicians, a new building for female nurses and employees was named for Dr. Nathaniel Emmons Paine. Paine Hall was completed and occupied in 1936. (Courtesy Westborough Public Library.)

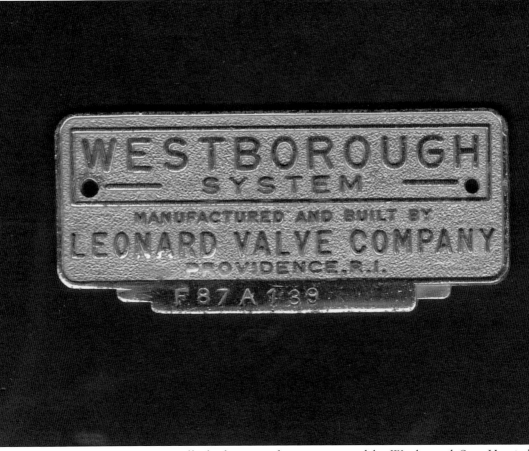

Given the great importance of hydrotherapy in the treatment model at Westborough State Hospital, superintendent Dr. Lang was actively involved in studying the continuous flow systems at the hospital and working to improve the actual process by which the therapy was administered. In 1933, he developed newer more precise controls for the system and had them patented. In honor of both the superintendent and the hospital, the new controls were called the Westborough System of Continuous Bath Control and were then mass produced for use on bath systems in other asylums. This equipment tag comes from a continuous bath system at the nearby Grafton State Hospital. (Courtesy Katherine Anderson.)

Four

LIFE AT WESTBOROUGH

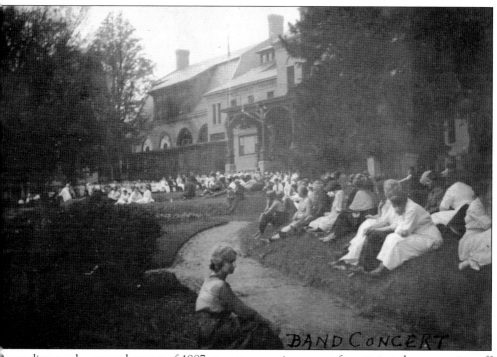

BAND CONCERT

According to the annual report of 1887, nurses were given one afternoon and one evening off
per week. Initially, it seems, they were allowed to go outside after the patients went to bed at 8:00
p.m. but lost the privilege after they were found to be mingling with the male attendants "under
questionable circumstances." Dr. Paine noted, perhaps wryly, that this behavior had gotten some
of these nurses previously discharged, and the same behavior "got them sacked" from Westborough
as well. (Courtesy Westborough Public Library.)

Westborough Training School for Nurses

CONNECTED WITH

THE WESTBOROUGH INSANE HOSPITAL

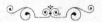

Graduating Exercises

NOVEMBER 4, 1891

"The second causes took the swift command,
The medicinal head, the ready hand;
All but eternal doom was conquered by their art."

The annual report of 1891 opens with a brief mention of improvement in the corps of nursing due to the "efficient training" of nurses, which had been started informally in 1889 and made a permanent fixture by 1890. The Westborough Training School for Nurses was made a permanent fixture, and the first class graduated on November 4, 1891. For the first six months after graduation, nurses wore a white cap and white apron over a calico dress. After six months, they transitioned to a blue-and-white striped dress. Both Dr. Paine and Dr. Adams served as instructors in the program. (Both, courtesy Massachusetts Department of Mental Health.)

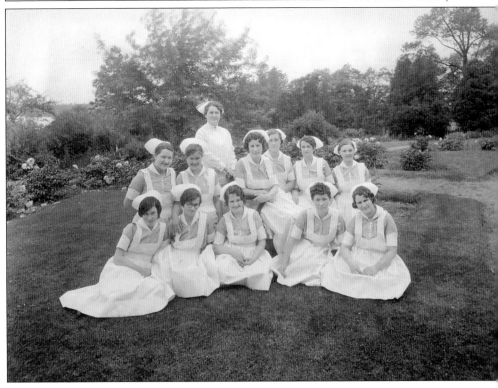

Two textbooks were prepared for the nursing course: *A Manual of Nursing*, originally written for the nurses attached to Bellevue Hospital in New York City, and *How to Care for the Insane* by Dr. William D. Granger. On graduation, nurses were awarded this certificate of completion. In the first year, nine women and three men graduated from the course. (Courtesy Massachusetts Department of Mental Health.)

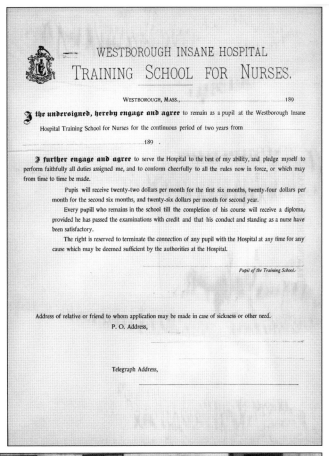

WESTBOROUGH INSANE HOSPITAL

TRAINING SCHOOL FOR NURSES.

WESTBOROUGH, MASS., _____189

I the undersigned, hereby engage and agree to remain as a pupil at the Westborough Insane Hospital Training School for Nurses for the continuous period of two years from

_____189 .

I further engage and agree to serve the Hospital to the best of my ability, and pledge myself to perform faithfully all duties assigned me, and to conform cheerfully to all the rules now in force, or which may from time to time be made.

Pupis will receive twenty-two dollars per month for the first six months, twenty-four dollars per month for the second six months, and twenty-six dollars per month for second year.

Every pupil who remains in the school till the completion of his course will receive a diploma, provided he has passed the examinations with credit and that his conduct and standing as a nurse have been satisfactory.

The right is reserved to terminate the connection of any pupil with the Hospital at any time for any cause which may be deemed sufficient by the authorities at the Hospital.

_____

Pupil of the Training School.

Address of relative or friend to whom application may be made in case of sickness or other need.

P. O. Address,

Telegraph Address,

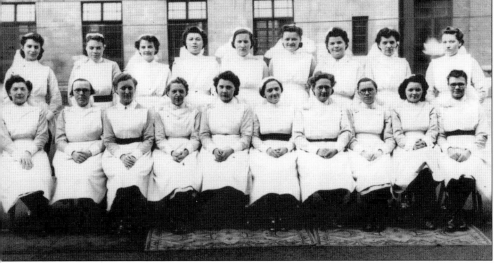

In the late 1880s, the nurses at Westborough State Hospital wore white caps and white aprons while male attendants wore blue flannel suits with brass buttons on the coat. The buttons bore the state arms. Nurses who attended the Westborough Training School were made to wear the badge of the school and a blue band on their caps. (Courtesy Massachusetts Department of Mental Health.)

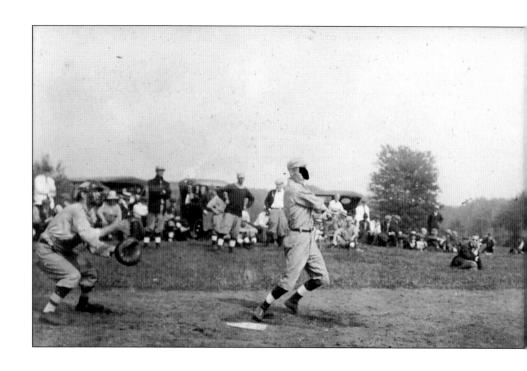

The patients' entertainment was well provided for with lectures, readings, concerts, and weekly dances. Plays were put on by local theater groups, and one annual report even mentions a magic show given by some of the hospital's medical staff. Religious services were held in the newly added chapel above the dining hall, led by neighborhood ministers. A traveling library was established, and collections of books were delivered regularly to the wards, chosen from the more than 600 volumes. The trustees even purchased a sailboat for use on Lake Chauncy. The patients had a private beach on the shore where they could swim and picnic during the summer months. (Both, courtesy Massachusetts Department of Mental Health.)

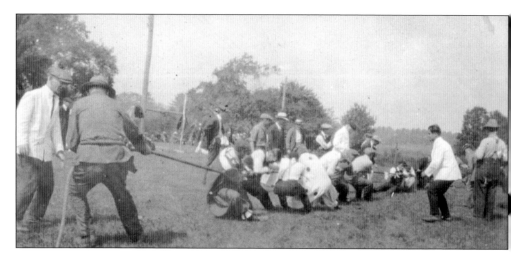

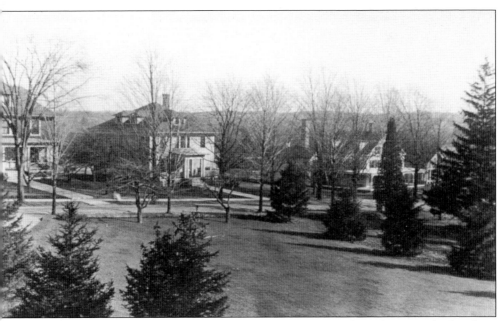

In spite of generous benefits—two weeks of paid vacation, an extra day off per month after three successful months of employment, and room and board—Westborough State Hospital had a great deal of difficulty with staff turnover. Some nurses left without notice or reason; others proved themselves unprepared for working with the insane. (Courtesy Westborough Public Library.)

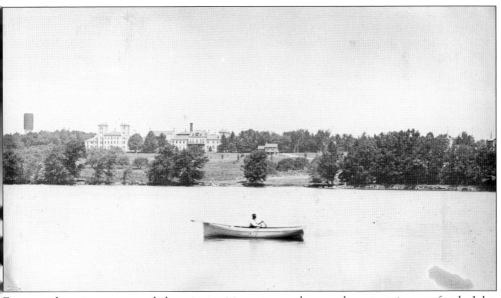

Frequent donations were made by private citizens to supplement the entertainment funds. John Felt Osgood was one of the hospital's most generous benefactors, giving hundreds of dollars each fiscal year for magic shows, theater productions, gym equipment, and games. After his passing in 1893, his wife, Elizabeth, continued his generosity, and the Osgood Cottage was officially named in his honor. (Courtesy Phil Kittredge.)

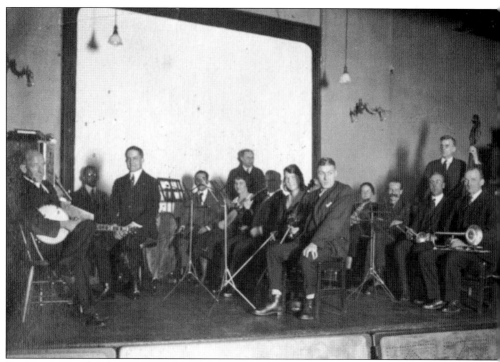

Entertainment for the patients included a weekly dance, at which the music was provided by a 15-piece band of both employees and patients. Music was also provided during lunches in the main dining hall. A moving picture booth was installed at the rear of the chapel, and a portable "moving picture apparatus" showed movies in various buildings. A traveling patient library of nearly 2,000 volumes circulated throughout the wards and included books, magazines, and newspapers, many of which were donated. Field days were held annually on the Fourth of July and Labor Day, and patients were taken to Worcester to see the Ringling Brothers Circus. The patients formed a baseball team that played against state hospital teams at Grafton, Medfield, and Worcester. (Above, courtesy Westborough Public Library; below, courtesy Massachusetts Department of Mental Health.)

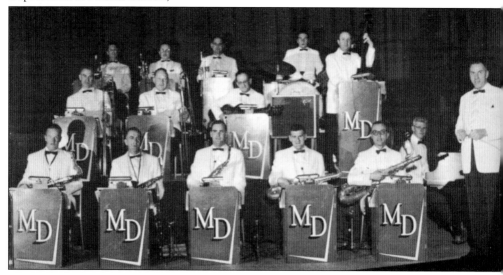

Westborough State Hospital also maintained an extensive medical library that housed volumes on the study of psychiatry and homeopathy, as well as scores of medical journals from around the world. Each time a volume was received by the library, each medical officer signed off on the addition of the volume or periodical. (Courtesy Ethan Dexter.)

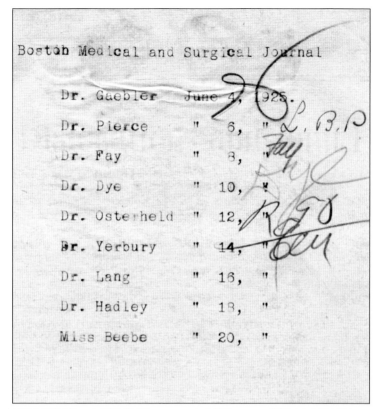

```
Boston Medical and Surgical Journal

    Dr. Gaebler      June 4, 1925.

    Dr. Pierce         "    6,   "

    Dr. Fay            "    8,   "

    Dr. Dye            "   10,   "

    Dr. Osterheld      "   12,   "

    Dr. Yerbury        "   14,   "

    Dr. Lang           "   16,   "

    Dr. Hadley         "   18,   "

    Miss Beebe         "   20,   "
```

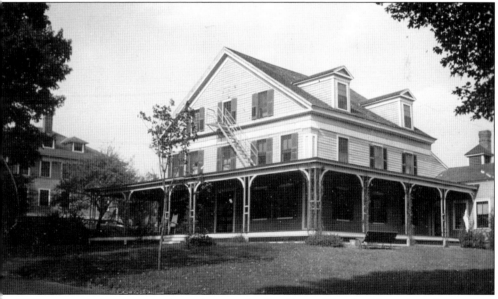

In 1920, appropriations were made to clear out the first floor of Stanley House in order to create a recreation room for the employees. The space was comfortably furnished with a piano and "facilities for letter writing." In 1921, the trustees reported that the "result justifies in every way the expenditure," as the employees used the space constantly and were "very appreciative of their privileges." (Courtesy Massachusetts Department of Mental Health.)

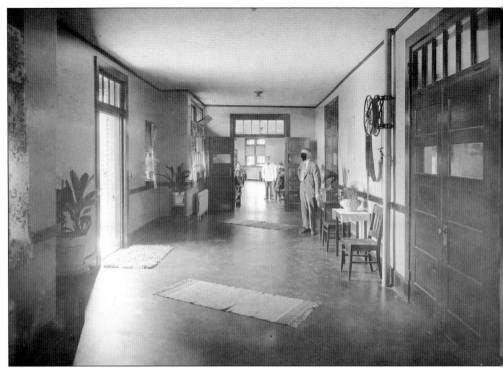

Over the course of the early 1900s, every effort was made to make the wards as comfortable as possible for the patients. Small comforts such as plants, decorations, and furniture were given a great deal of thought and attention. The wards were visited twice each day by a physician who was able to check in on each patient as he made his rounds, as the patient-to-physician ratio was kept exceedingly low. A new occupational therapy room was added in the main hospital building in order to provide a more comfortable, better-lit space for patients to complete their work. (Both, courtesy Massachusetts Department of Mental Health.)

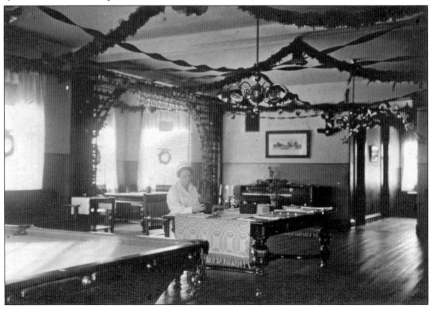

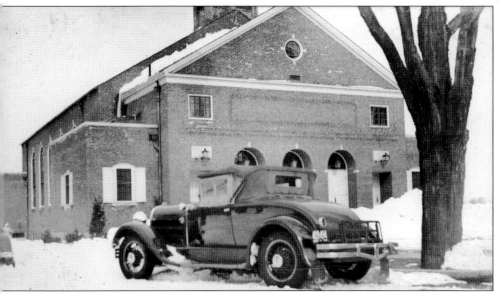

In order to further assist in funding patient activities, Dr. Lang created a canteen that sold snacks, drinks, and sundries. The money helped pay for dances, games, and music plus bus rides, picnics, suppers, and dances. As the entertainment budget grew, it was clear that a larger space was needed for gatherings and performances. The current hall above the dining room that doubled as a chapel could only hold 300 people if they were packed in elbow to elbow. The room could only be reached by two narrow wooden staircases and was considered a safety hazard. The trustees proposed the building of a separate assembly hall, and work began in 1931. (Above, courtesy Massachusetts Department of Mental Health; below, courtesy Westborough Public Library.)

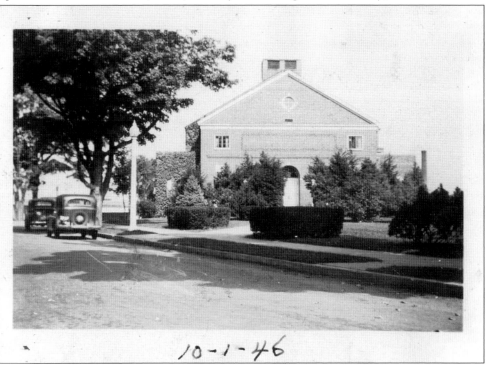

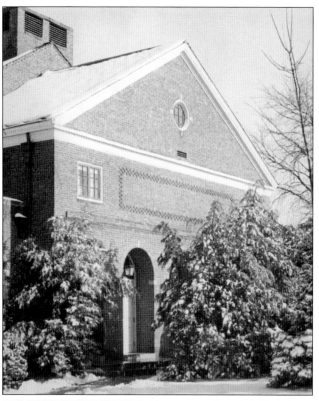

The 1,000-seat assembly hall was completed and opened for use in October 1931. The lower floor of the hall housed a recreation room, a bowling alley, the canteen, and a serving room for events. Named for the superintendent, Lang Auditorium played host to a number of performances, including community theater, traveling magic shows, and talent shows. The auditorium hosted the graduation ceremonies for the hospital's nursing program as well as weekly religious services. The hospital formed its own orchestra and chorus, and the portable moving picture machine was put to use in the new auditorium. Employee dances and socials were also held regularly in the hall. (Both, courtesy Massachusetts Department of Mental Health.)

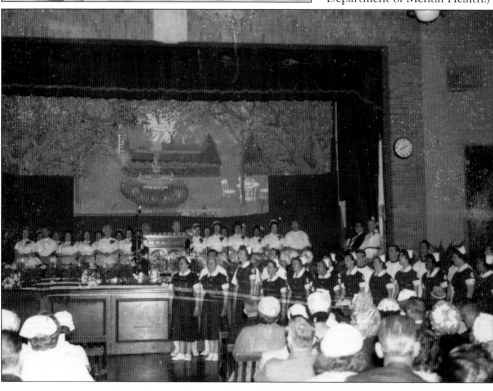

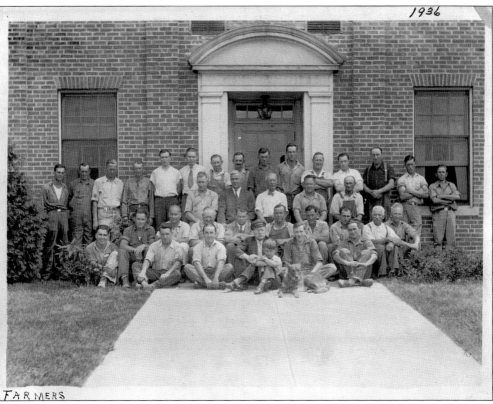

FARMERS

The above image from 1936 was taken in front of the Farm Dormitory. The head farmer, Raymond L. Whitney (also pictured below), and his team of farmers was responsible for a multitude of crops such as potatoes, asparagus, cauliflower, and spinach as well as pears, tomatoes, and summer squash. The 1936 season saw the highest quantity of pork production since the farm's beginnings, even though Whitney considered the crop production disappointing. The early spring and cold, wet weather contributed to a less than stellar yield, though the 807,936 pounds of milk production may have made up for the poor growing season. That year, Westborough State Hospital donated 30 cows to other Massachusetts institutions. (Both, courtesy Westborough Public Library.)

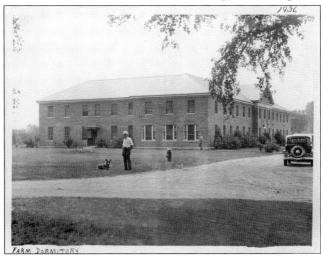

FARM DORMITORY

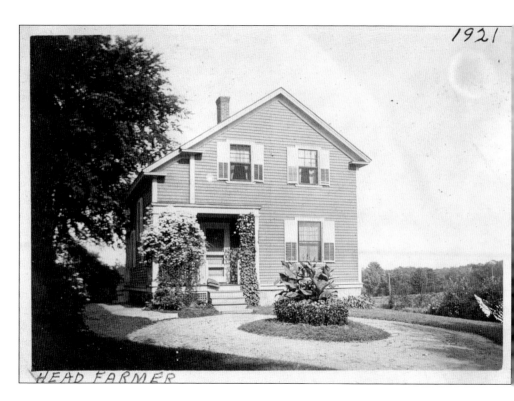

The head farmer lived in a small cottage on campus, which was very similar in design to Osgood Cottage. It is located directly next to the assistant superintendent's house and is known as Houghton House, which is the oldest extant building on the state hospital campus. Houghton House was built around 1820 and predates the creation of the reform school. Stanley House, which was acquired along with its attendant farmland in the early 1890s for the price of $8,000 for a time housed the head engineer as well as the male kitchen and engine room staff. The house was demolished in September 1949. (Both, courtesy Westborough Public Library.)

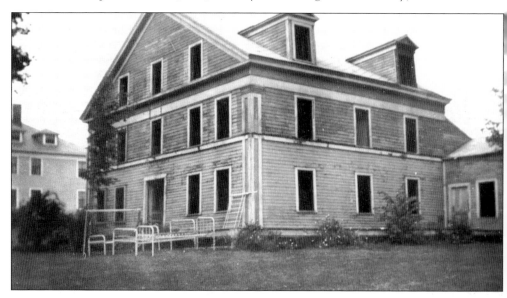

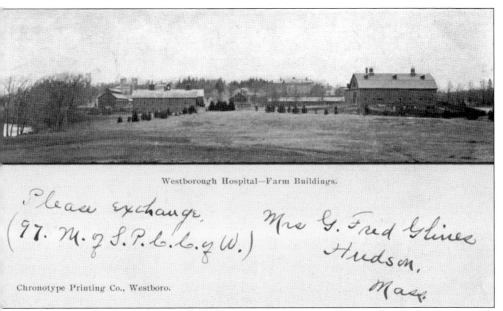

Westborough Hospital—Farm Buildings.

Please exchange,
(97. M. of S.P.C.C. of W.)

Mrs. G. Fred Glines
Hudson,
Mass.

Chronotype Printing Co., Westboro.

Over the years, the farm expanded as the hospital acquired a number of the surrounding family farms. Some of the barns on the property were original to the reform school, but most were built by the hospital. Pictured above are the hay barns and dairy barns that would later be destroyed by fire. Below is an image of the piggery, which was the same size as the administration building and housed more than 1,000 pigs. It, too, would be lost to fire and never rebuilt to that scale again. However, the hospital became known for its pork production as well as its high volume of milk production. (Above, courtesy Phil Kittredge; below, courtesy Massachusetts Department of Mental Health.)

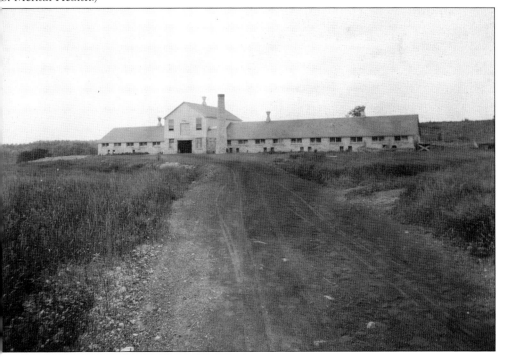

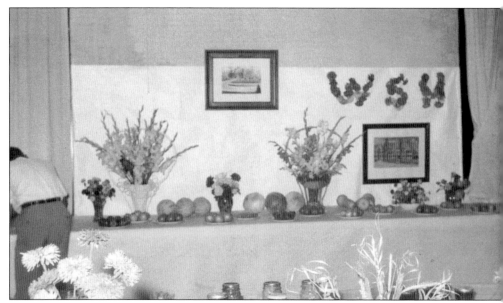

The farm at Westborough State Hospital produced enough fruit, vegetables, meat, eggs, and milk that they were able to supply other state institutions with goods and even allow the patients to sell some of the produce to the public and to the staff in the hospital's canteen. The dairy herd produced nearly 400,000 quarts of milk annually, which supported the patients' milk-heavy diet. It was believed that balanced, nutrition-rich diets aided in curing acute cases of mental illness. Along with the rest cure, the milk diet was very popular in the early years of the hospital. (Above, courtesy Westborough Public Library; below, courtesy Massachusetts Department of Mental Health.)

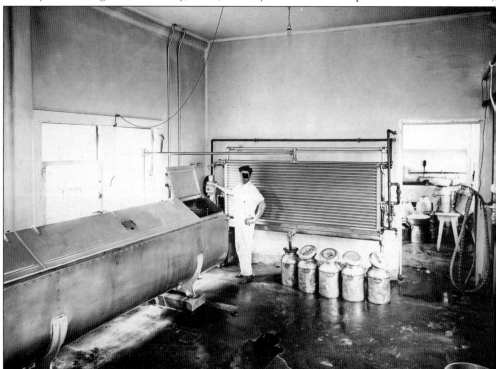

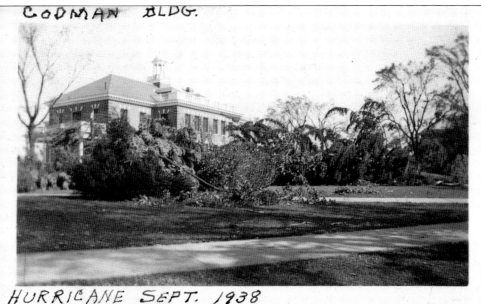

CODMAN BLDG.

HURRICANE SEPT. 1938

On September 21, 1939, "the unique event of the year occurred" when a hurricane struck New England. The storm caused a great deal of damage to the hospital campus, tearing off portions of roof coverings, uprooting trees, and demolishing some of the smaller outbuildings. One entire section of the roof on the main building was torn away, and the slates were ripped from the roof of Paine Hall. The kitchen exhaust ventilator on the Farm Dormitory was blown away as were the doors on the Heath barn. Electricity went out as well as telegraph communications. The storm damaged crops, and the grounds were also heavily damaged. Dr. Lang remarked in the annual report that the grounds were so ruined that familiar landmarks were no longer, while new vistas were revealed. (Courtesy Westborough Public Library.)

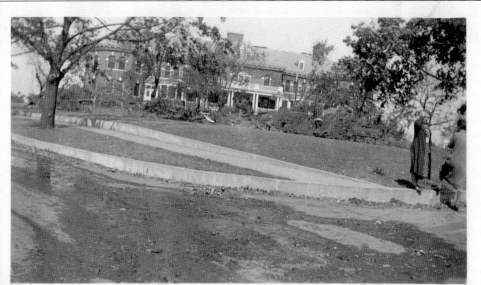

TALBOT BLDG.   SEPT. 1938.

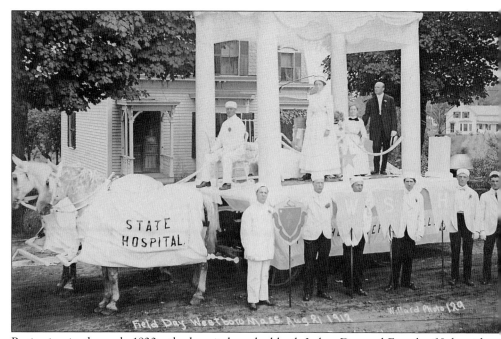

Beginning in the early 1920s, the hospital marked both Labor Day and Fourth of July with an annual field day where patients, staff, and guests played games, ran races, and picnicked on the main lawn of the hospital. The above image is of the 1947 celebration. Below is a similar view of the celebration held in 1951. The hospital celebration often overlapped with the town celebration, allowing the patients to participate in town activities as well. The field day tradition carried on until the late 1950s, when presumably, the ballooning patient population and declining staff population, coupled with the use of medication, made the field-day activities impossible to supervise appropriately. (Above, courtesy Phil Kittredge; below, courtesy Westborough Public Library.)

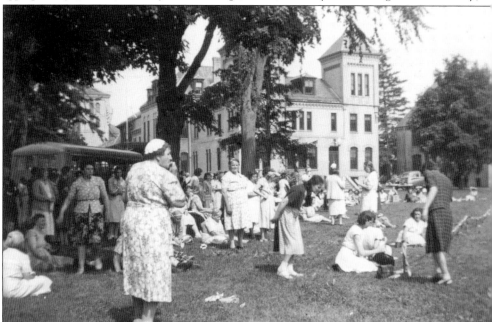

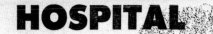

HOSPITAL DAY

"The Mentally Ill Can Come Back"

WESTBOROUGH STATE HOSPITAL

APRIL 30, 1958

1:30 P.M. TO 4:00 P.M.

DO COME AND BRING A FRIEND

PROGRAM OF ACTIVITIES

EXHIBITS - GUIDED TOURS - MOTION PICTURES

PRESENTATION OF SERVICE PINS TO VOLUNTEERS

A good deal of work was done on the campus of Westborough State Hospital by community volunteers. These volunteers worked in nearly every department at the hospital but played the largest part in the recreation department. They aided in planning almost every event on campus as well as trips to town, bus trips to the circus, and other off-campus events. The volunteers were honored annually at an open house, where they were presented with awards and given pins marking their volunteer service. The public was welcomed, and the event drew as many as 700 visitors. (Courtesy Massachusetts Department of Mental Health.)

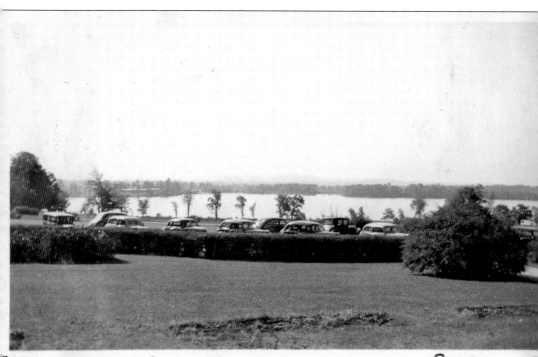

SOUTH FROM ADM. BLDG.   SEPT. 19

The annual report of 1932 refers to 50 years prior to the opening of Westborough Insane Hospital when hospitals gave more thought to the custody of the insane than to their treatment. Patients were being restrained either chemically or mechanically, and treatment was largely experimental. The trustees noted that "additional buildings are not so desirable as more cures." Treatment should be the study rather than confinement, and hospitals should focus on these by engaging in research into trauma and recovery, as well as working to employ new methods while decreasing the use of treatments such as wet packs and fever therapies. Throughout the early 20th century, Westborough worked to take the lead in asylum medicine. (Courtesy Westborough Public Library.)

Five

A New Era

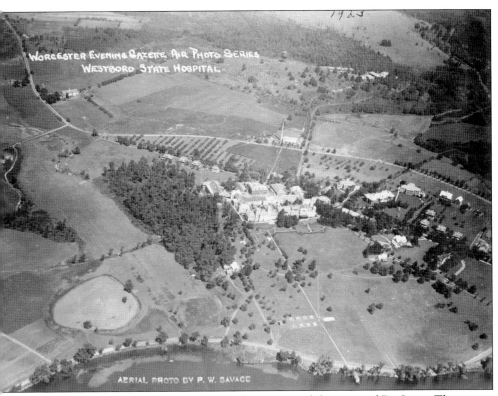

Westborough weathered World War II under the continued direction of Dr. Lang. The census peaked at nearly 2,000 patients, and 156 deaths were recorded. Dr. N. Emmons Paine declined to continue as a trustee, and a great number of staff again enlisted in the armed forces. Lang remarked in the annual report of 1942 that "the outlook for the future is not bright." (Courtesy Westborough Public Library.)

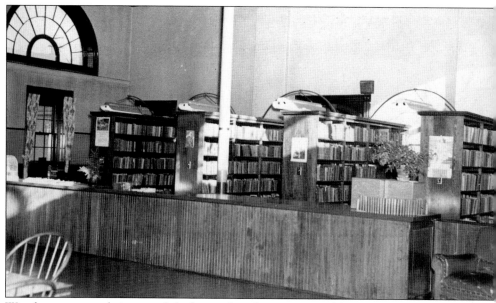

War shortages greatly impacted the hospital, making it impossible to request appropriations. In order to fill some of the staffing vacancies, patients were drafted to help out on the wards. In spite of these shortages, the patient library grew substantially each year until 1942, when it was moved into the space previously occupied by the congregate dining room. By then, the library held 2,42_ volumes and 108 magazine subscriptions. (Courtesy Massachusetts Department of Mental Health.

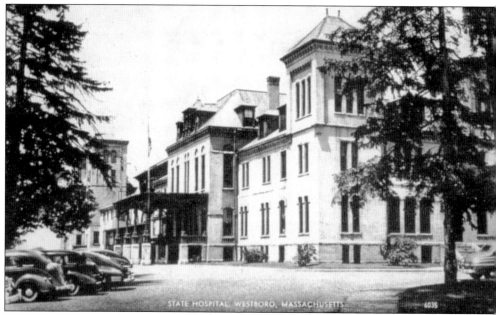

The early 1940s brought about a major change in treatment as electroconvulsive therapy (ECT) grew in popularity. Developed in Italy in the late 1930s, ECT made use of electricity to induce seizures in a patient as doctors mistakenly believed that epilepsy and schizophrenia could not exist in one body. Coupled with psychotherapy, ECT became a staple of treatment at Westborough well into the 1950s. (Courtesy Westborough Public Library.)

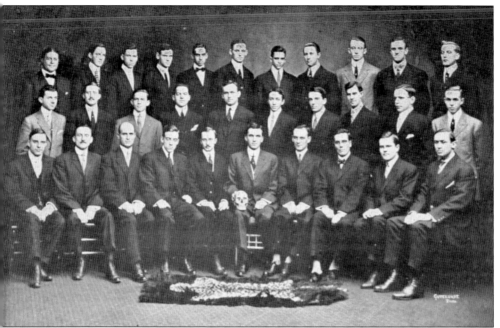

As World War II drew to a close, Dr. Lang retired as superintendent in 1946 after nearly 30 years at Westborough. He was succeeded by his assistant, Dr. Rollin V. Hadley. Though the war was over, it remained difficult to get supplies. Some vacancies were filled on the wards, but the staff numbers did not immediately return to normal. Farm labor was scarce still, and the nurses' training school was forced to close on November 13, 1946, due to declining enrollment. The iris pictured here is labeled "Dr. Hadley's Iris 1936." It likely grew in the yard of the assistant superintendent's cottage, where Dr. Hadley resided until his promotion 10 years later. (Above, courtesy John Gray; below, courtesy Massachusetts Department of Mental Health.)

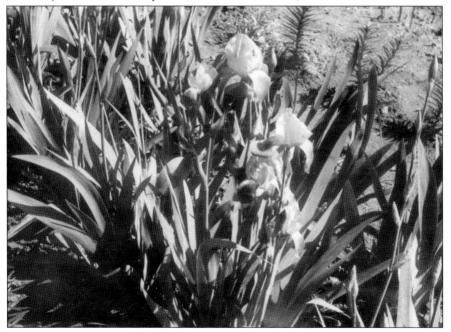

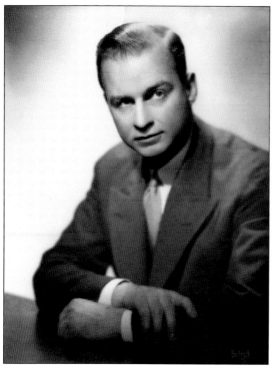

In February 1944, Dr. Perry Baird, a prominent Boston physician, suffered a breakdown and was taken by police from his home in Chestnut Hill to Westborough State Hospital. Dr. Baird had been so respected as a physician that Dr. Lang himself had called Baird's home to arrange his admission to the hospital. It was not the first time Dr. Baird had entered treatment, but it was the most salient. Over the course of his time at Westborough, Dr. Baird recorded each experience and encounter with doctors, orderlies, and other patients. His account is often bleak and torturous; his treatment was best described as "barbaric at worst and cold at best." (Both, courtesy Mimi Baird.)

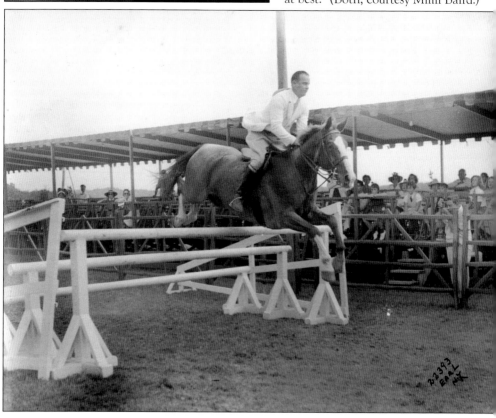

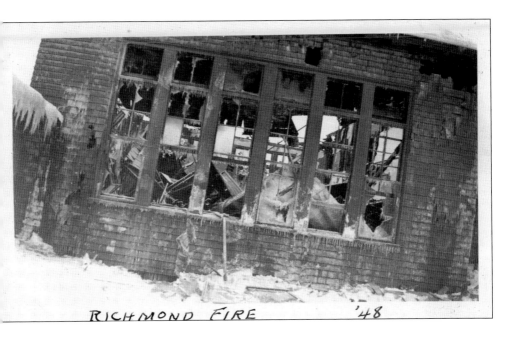

RICHMOND FIRE   '48

Fires in the colony buildings were common and often caused a great deal of damage. In the early 1920s, the boiler was damaged by fire and on the verge of collapse. In 1922, the interiors of Speare and Dewson were renovated to increase fire safety. Eventually, most of the electrical system was also updated to prevent fire. On January 28, 1948, a fire ripped through the Richmond Colony on the southwestern shore of Lake Chauncy. A separate sanitarium for men with tuberculosis was the only building that survived the fire and continued to be used to house tuberculosis patients. The fire-damaged buildings remained vacant until they were demolished in 1957. (Courtesy Westborough Public Library.)

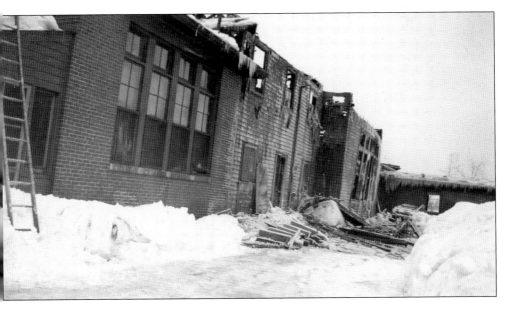

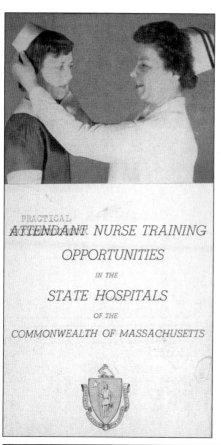

PRACTICAL
ATTENDANT NURSE TRAINING
OPPORTUNITIES
IN THE
STATE HOSPITALS
OF THE
COMMONWEALTH OF MASSACHUSETTS

Four years after the closing of the nurses' training school, Westborough revived the program by creating a new attendant nurses' training school, a 15-month program that would then allow nurses to transfer to other institutions after receiving their certificate. Nurses studied not just psychiatric nursing but general practical nursing as well. In spite of the success of the training school, the state hospital continually struggled with staff shortages on the nursing staff. They had difficulty hiring qualified nurses, and many of their graduates moved on to other institutions, including general hospitals, as the program was not specifically focused on psychiatric nursing. (Both, courtesy Massachusetts Department of Mental Health.)

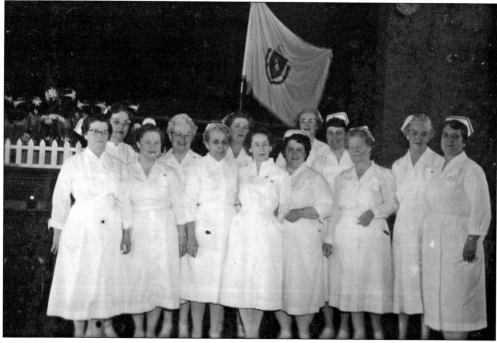

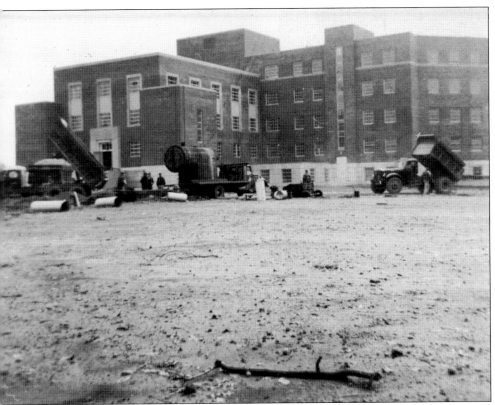

In April 1950, the hospital broke ground on a $1.6 million tuberculosis building on the opposite side of Lyman Street. The building was completed and dedicated in 1952, named for retiring superintendent Dr. Rollin Hadley. The building alleviated some of the overcrowding at the main hospital and filled the need for tuberculosis treatment left by the abandonment of the Richmond Colony. While the building filled a great need on the state hospital campus, it also presented immediate problems. There were repairs needed almost immediately when "unforeseen defects and omissions" were discovered. Additionally, many of the patients who were moved to Hadley were found to be in need of immediate surgery because of the seriousness of tuberculosis infection. (Courtesy Westborough Public Library.)

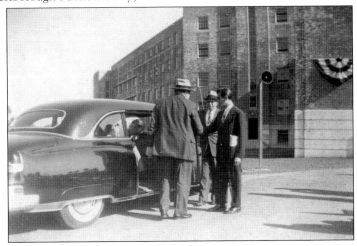

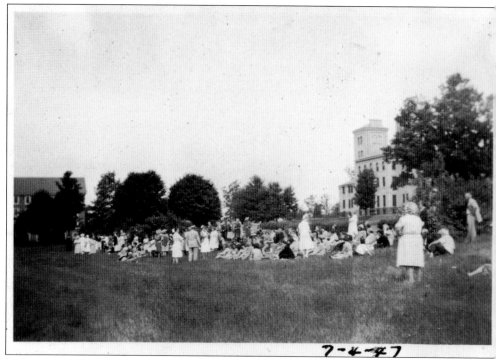

By the close of the 1951 fiscal year, there were 1,724 patients in the hospital. Overcrowding remained a major issue that was especially compounded by the number of chronic alcoholics and elderly on the wards. The medical staff was closely monitoring the efficacy of both electroconvulsive therapy and lobotomy in the chronic patients, and they found that, by and large, both treatment were providing relief for most patients, though the lobotomy was only used as a last resort. Despite the steadily growing patient population, recreation and entertainment opportunities remained a priority. A number of community organizations helped to supplement the entertainment offering by putting on plays, concerts, and variety shows. (Both, courtesy Westborough Public Library.)

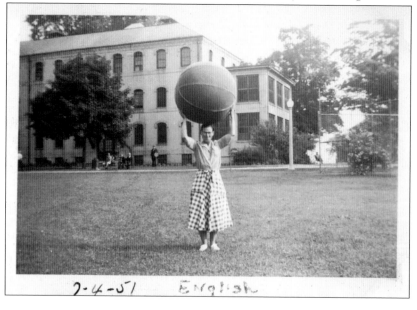

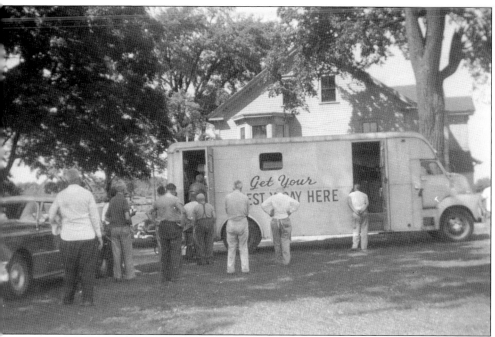

In the early 1850s, one in four individuals died from pulmonary tuberculosis, a highly infectious bacterial disease that infected the lungs. Commonly called "consumption" because of rapid weight loss caused by the illness, the hallmark of tuberculosis infection was a chronic cough that produced blood. Because tuberculosis is so easily spread through the air by way of a cough, sneeze, or other transmission of spit, patients who were infected needed to be quarantined. Given the rapid rate at which this disease was transmitted, it was often discovered as a complicating factor in many cases of insanity and was therefore often treated in hospitals for the insane. A tuberculosis diagnosis is most often based on a chest x-ray. Though Westborough had their own x-ray machines, they also provided mobile clinics in order to screen all patients and employees. (Both, courtesy Westborough Public Library.)

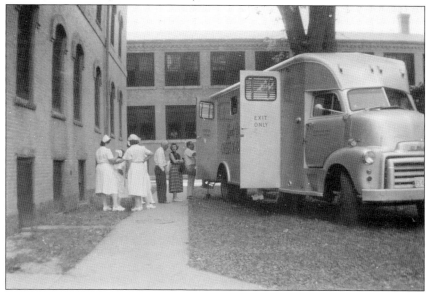

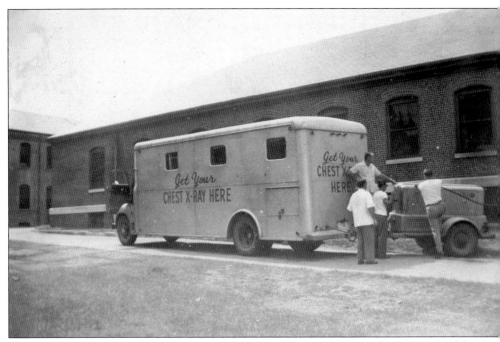

Early treatments for tuberculosis included a strict regimen of bed rest, fresh air, a healthy diet and a gradual increase in activity levels—all of which fit well with the homeopathic treatment model at Westborough. By the early 1950s, a tuberculosis vaccine had been developed and tested which dramatically reduced the instances of infection, but the vaccine was only made available in the UK as doctors in the United States had been unable to replicate their results. Instead, hospitals continued to practice quarantine measures and treat the infection with rest and fresh air. Vaccines for tuberculosis are still not widely available, though it has been proven that vaccination and early treatment of active cases are the only way to prevent the spread of the disease. (Both courtesy Westborough Public Library.)

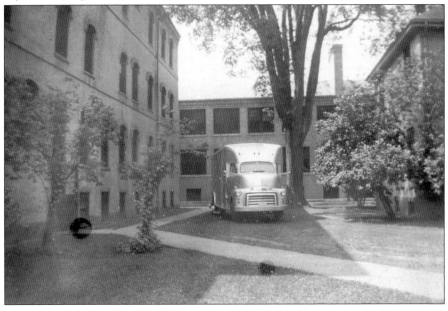

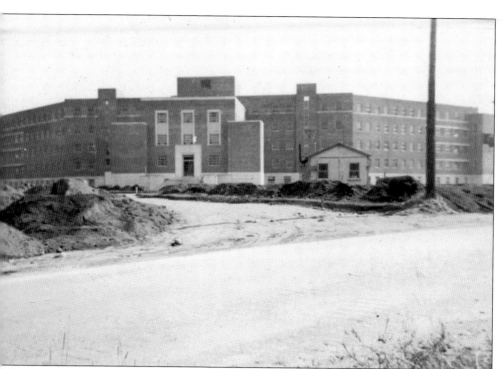

Tuberculosis (TB) appeared to occur more often in those who were already diagnosed as mentally ill, leading to a larger-than-average number of active TB patients in the asylums. At first, these patients were simply separated from the general patient population, as the rest cure (which was the most common treatment for TB) was already being used at Westborough, but it eventually became necessary to expand the treatment model for TB patients up to and including surgeries. The Hadley Building had a state-of-the-art x-ray machine that was used to perform routine chest x-rays for both employees and patients. The annual report from 1953 noted that there was a greater number of men receiving treatment than women. (Courtesy Westborough Public Library.)

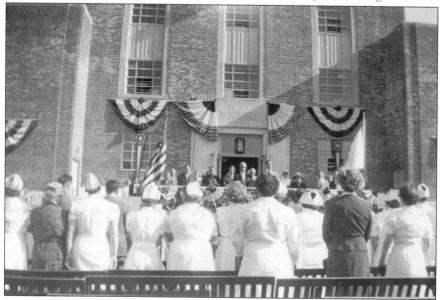

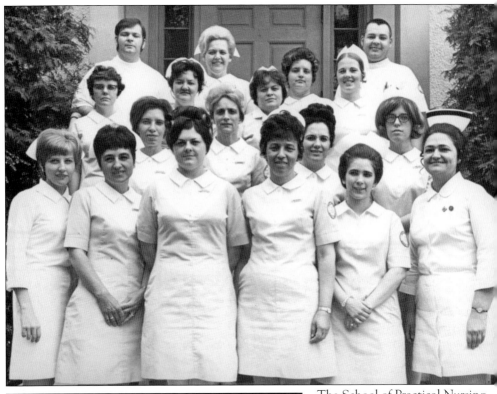

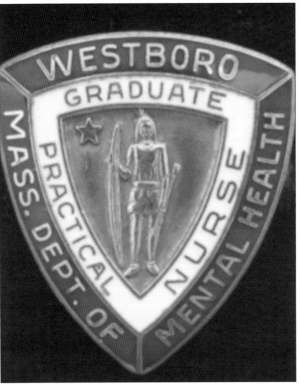

The School of Practical Nursing continued to graduate students well into the late 1950s under the direction of Gertrude Poskitt, RN. The program had previously been affiliated with Tewksbury State Hospital but shifted to Worcester City Hospital, presumably in order to broaden practical experience. In 1956 Westborough State Hospital was approved for training psychiatric residents as well as clinical training in occupational therapy and social services. The annual report of 1957 notes that a new skeleton was purchased for the nursing school as well as a stove. Throughout the 1960s, the school of practical nursing continued to turn out top graduates, though the hospital still struggled with employee turnover in the nursing department. (Above, courtesy Massachusetts Department of Mental Health; left, courtesy Phil Kittredge.)

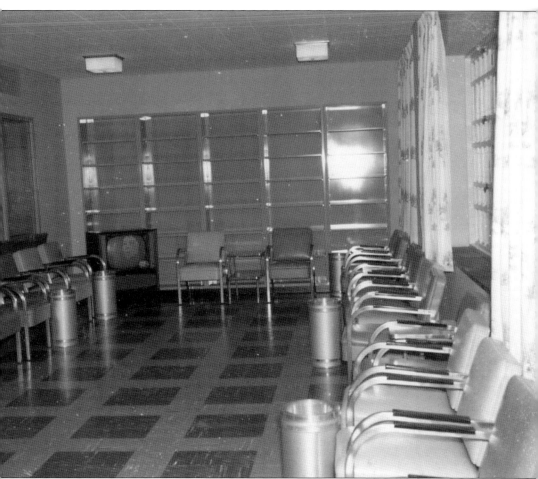

The next major shift in treatment was the advent of the prefrontal lobotomy. In the early 1950s, the medical staff began exploring the effectiveness of psychosurgery on patients for whom electroconvulsive therapy was not working. According to the annual report, "no patient is made worse by the surgery," but still, lobotomy was only relied upon as a last resort. Despite this positive assertion, the medical staff continued to emphasize electroconvulsive therapy as the primary treatment method. By the late 1950s, the medical staff began consciously pairing electroconvulsive therapy with group and individual psychotherapy with an eye to decreasing the number of treatments needed. (Courtesy Massachusetts Department of Mental Health.)

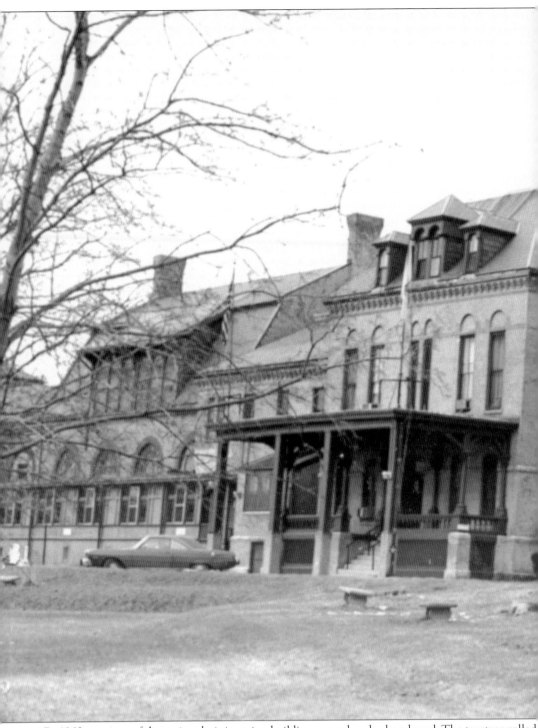

By 1960, portions of the main administration building were already abandoned. The trustees called for a plan to replace most of the buildings, citing the risk of fire hazard in the oldest buildings, many of which had been standing for almost a century. Codman and Childs were both closed to be renovated in the future, and a number of outbuildings were abandoned, including Dorm A

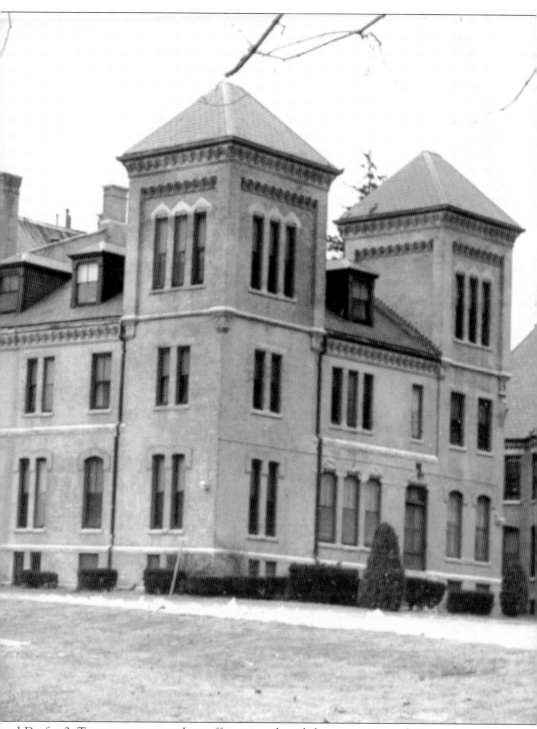

and Durfee 2. Turnover amongst the staff continued, and the vacancies made it necessary to decrease the number of patients participating in industrial therapy and grounds work. (Courtesy Westborough Public Library.)

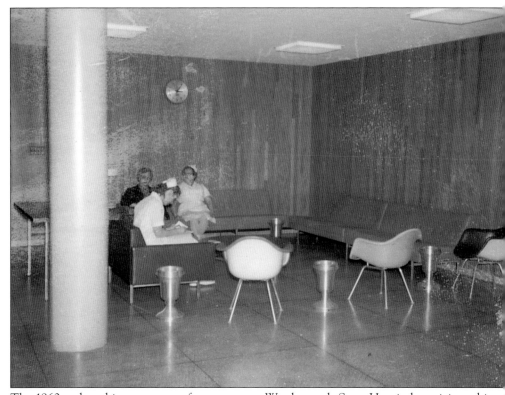

The 1960s ushered in a new era of treatment as Westborough State Hospital participated in a research study on the value of antidepressants versus electroconvulsive therapy. There was a marked increase in both ECT and the prescribing of medications to all patients at the hospital. Most of the staff was focused on providing as much treatment as possible to new admissions, hoping to increase the number of discharges. (Courtesy Massachusetts Department of Mental Health.)

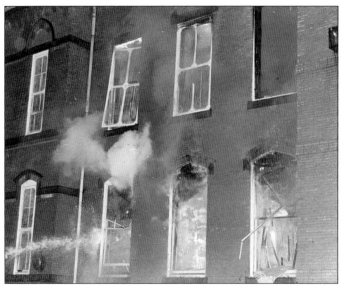

Sometime in the mid-1950s, there was a large fire in the wards behind the main administration building, the damage from which was never repaired. The same wards caught fire again in 1975 and were simply boarded up. A number of firefighters were thrown from the building while fighting the fire when the roof collapsed. Thankfully, it was winter, and they landed in the snow. Both fires were ultimately listed as suspicious. (Courtesy Phil Kittredge.)

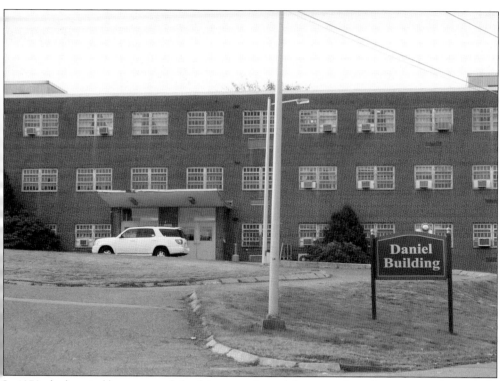

In 1970, the hospital began to scale back its operations. A large number of programs such as sewing class were phased out, and the last class of nurses graduated from the School of Practical Nursing. The Warren Colony had already been closed to patients for several years and was turned over to the Department of Fisheries and Wildlife. The piggery was also phased out as farming activity decreased. There was a marked increase in the number of drug addicts and alcoholics admitted to the hospital, requiring that the hospital continue to lead both AA and Al-Anon meetings in the Talbot Building. (Above, courtesy Massachusetts Department of Mental Health; below, courtesy National Register of Historic Places.)

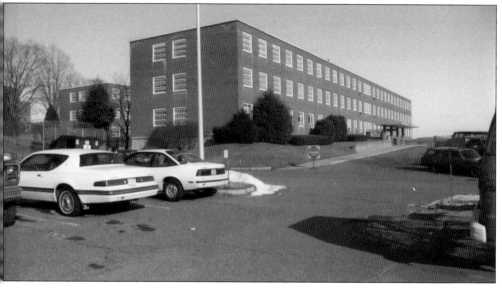

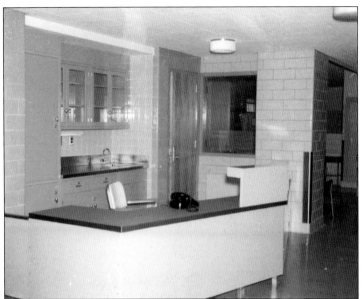

As the inpatient population was dramatically reduced, wards were closed down, some slated for demolition. The hospital's administrative structure was decentralized as unitization went into effect in April 1971. As of June 30, 1971, there were 1,100 patients in the hospital compared to a peak census of 2,500 in the early 1950s. (Courtesy Massachusetts Department of Mental Health.)

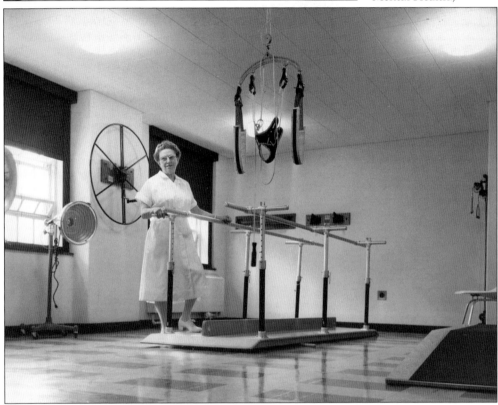

The hospital property totaled 604.45 acres at the close of 1971. Of 910 employees, 232 resigned as continued changes were made in the administrative structure of the hospital. E Building was closed as a patient residence with plans for possible renovation into a disturbed children's unit. That unit, the RFK Children's Action Corps, would eventually be located next to the administration building. (Courtesy Massachusetts Department of Mental Health.)

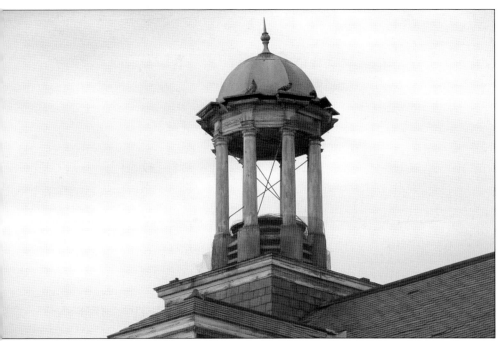

By the 1970s, there was a major focus on transferring geriatric patients into the community or into more appropriate placements. This dramatically decreased the inpatient population at Westborough and allowed for more efficient restructuring of the wards. In 2008, the Sharp Building, attached to the geriatric wards known as Hennessy and Daniels, was converted into a Department of Youth Services program as well and housed the regional offices for Central Massachusetts. The Daniels Building housed the only psychiatric unit specifically for deaf patients. (Both, courtesy Massachusetts Department of Mental Health.)

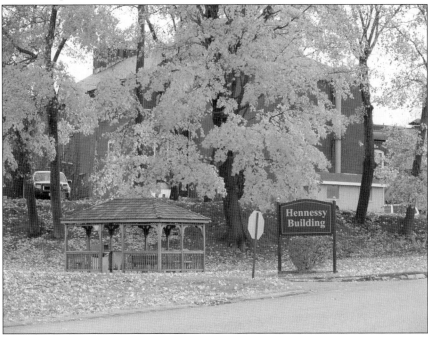

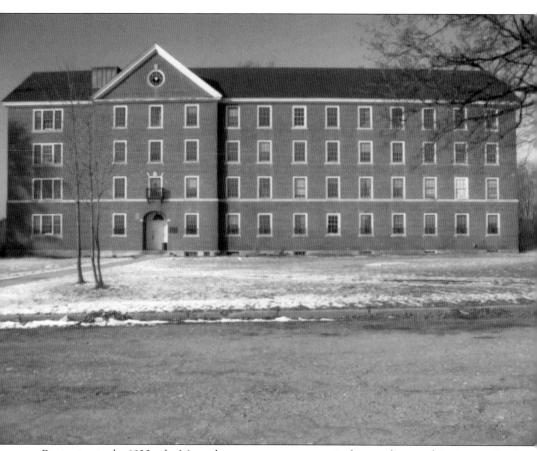

Beginning in the 1930s, the Massachusetts courts were required to conduct psychiatric examinations on juvenile offenders. These offenders were referred to Westborough State Hospital for "special examination and report." Eventually, the state hospital campus became home to a number of juvenile programs. Paine Hall, now Allen Hall, was left vacant for a number of years until the Robert F. Kennedy Action Corps moved its residential program from behind the wards to Paine Hall. The building was deemed unsafe, and the corps was forced to build a new building within the shell of the original Paine Hall. It currently houses a Department of Youth Services program. It was added to the National Register of Historic Places in 1993 with the rest of the buildings on the campus. (Courtesy National Register of Historic Places.)

Six

FAREWELL

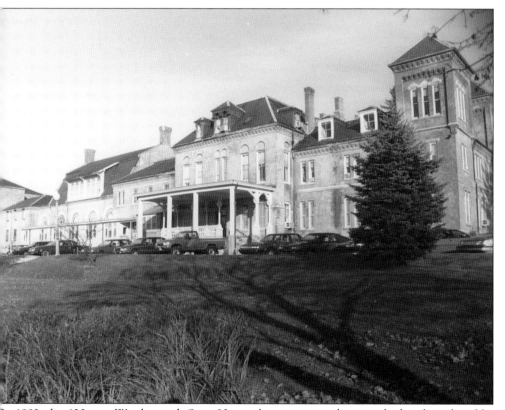

In 1993, the 600-acre Westborough State Hospital campus was photographed and cataloged by Candace Jenkins as part of the nomination process for the National Register of Historic Places. The property was added to the register a year later, and the buildings were granted historic status. The hospital remained open and operating until 2010. (Courtesy National Register of Historic Places.)

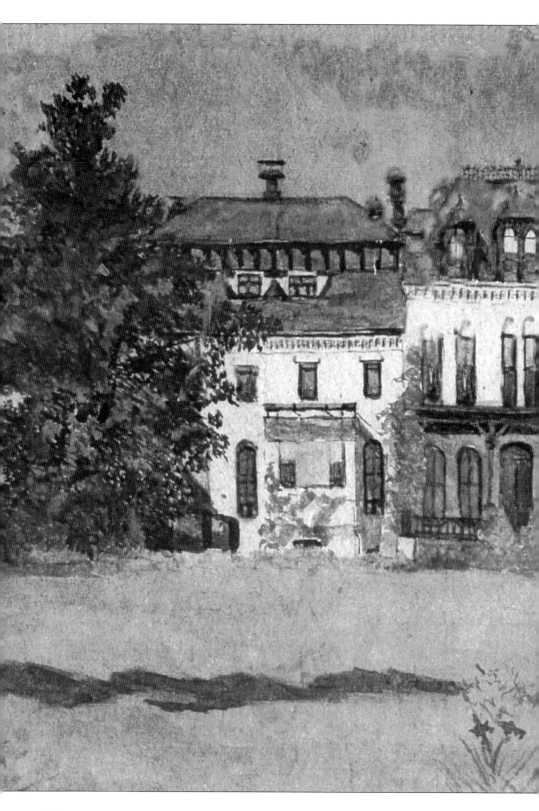

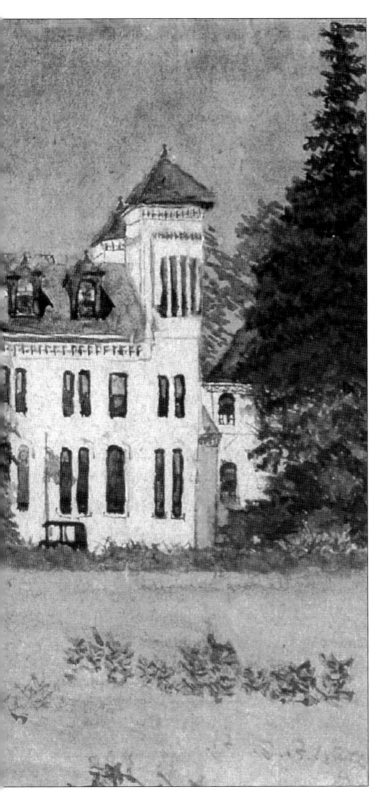

The Massachusetts Department of Mental Health announced in 2009 that it would be closing Westborough State Hospital by the end of the following year. Four years earlier, the state had decided to allocate funds for the building of a new facility in Worcester that would replace the aging state hospitals in both Westborough and Worcester. Originally, Westborough State Hospital was slated to remain open until the new Worcester facility was completed, but instead, the hospital closed two years before the official opening of the Worcester Recovery Center. The closure came on the heels of a nearly $70 million budget shortfall. (Courtesy Ethan Dexter)

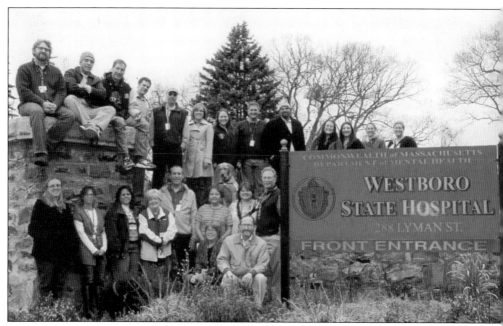

The announcement that Westborough State Hospital was to close came as a surprise, as the original plan had been for Westborough to remain open while a new facility was being constructed on the site of the former Worcester State Hospital. Instead, the state elected to save Westborough's $43 million budget by closing it early. (Courtesy Ethan Dexter.)

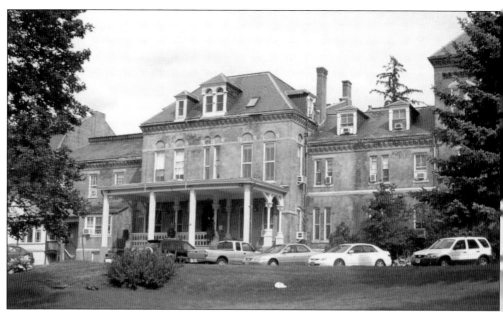

Admissions were frozen in August 2009 amidst protests from the remaining staff members. The first inpatient unit was converted to a community placement unit by December of that year, and the staff began working on transferring patients. Many of the remaining employees were laid off—some involuntarily, while others took incentives for voluntary layoff. (Courtesy Massachusetts Department of Mental Health.)

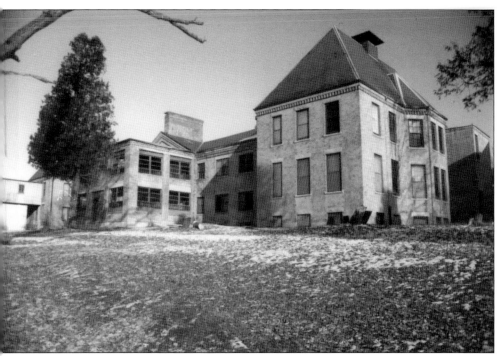

By the time closure was announced, a number of the wards had already been abandoned for many years. A massive collapse in Ward A destroyed all three floors of the wards, taking furniture, medical equipment, and filing cabinets full of paperwork with it. A large hole in the roof opened the century-old building up to the elements, warping the floors, making them spongy and unsafe. Multiple fires were reported in the abandoned wards, and the buildings became targets for scrappers and vandals. Though parts of the wards were boarded up, many of the windows and a number of doors remained open. (Both, courtesy National Register of Historic Places.)

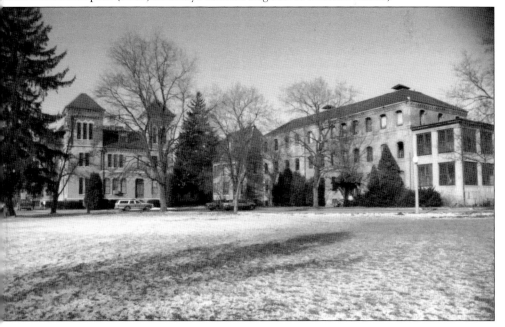

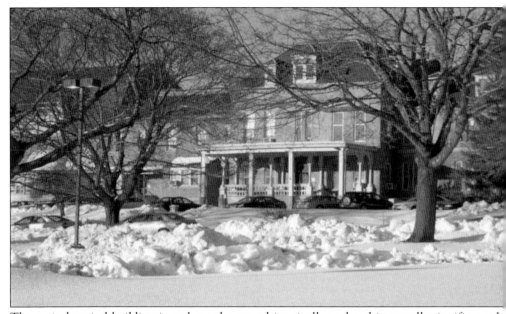

The main hospital building is perhaps the most historically and architecturally significant. It was designed in 1848 by Elias Carter and James Savage, then expanded in 1876 by Cutting and Holman of Worcester. Eventually, two of the towers that were most recognizable as part of the original reform school were dismantled at some point, likely due to age and probable decay. Other architectural features such as copper roofing and flashing, slate tiles, and wrought-iron can be seen on many of the buildings throughout the campus, including the former dead house, or morgue, which squats just behind the main building. (Above, courtesy Massachusetts Department of Mental Health; below, courtesy National Register of Historic Places.)

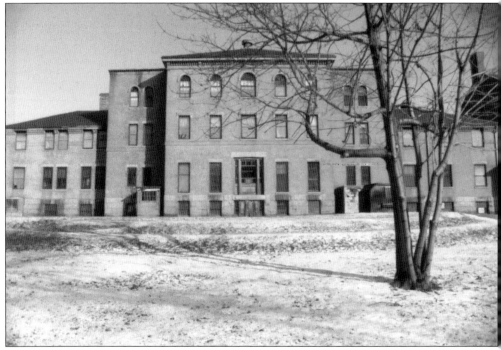

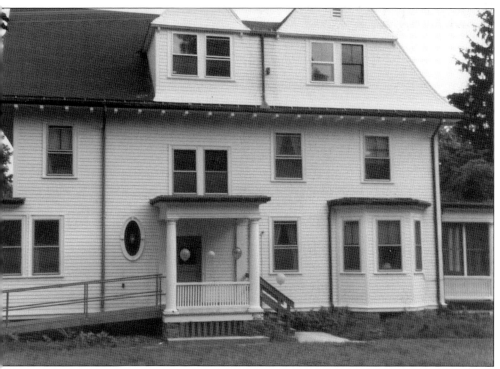

The Westborough State Hospital campus, with the exception of Allen Hall (Paine Hall) and the Sharp Building, remained abandoned until the fall of 2018 when Pulte Homes began demolition on the campus. Beginning with Osgood Cottage, which still sat overlooking Lake Chancy, crews moved quickly, abating and demolishing the house in one day. Crews then moved to abate the superintendent's cottage along with three of the nurses' houses on Hospital Road at the edge of the campus. A fenced-in area to the right of the main hospital building served as a dump site for the majority of the construction debris. (Both, courtesy National Register of Historic Places.)

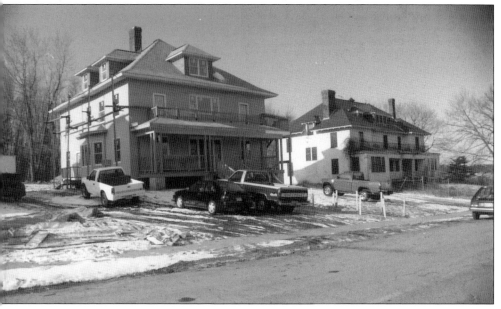

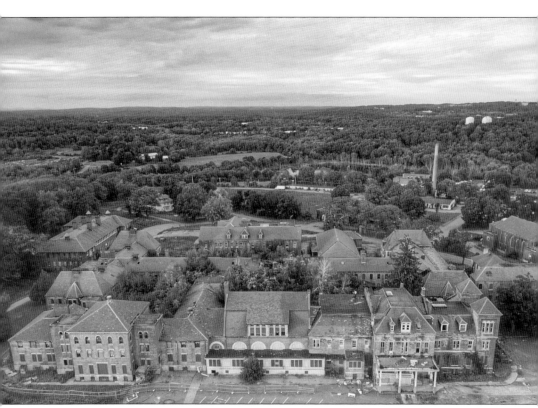

Following the closure of the hospital, the town negotiated the purchase of 95 of the 600 acres with the Division of Capital Asset Management and Maintenance; the sale was finalized in 2014. Under the agreement with the state, the town purchased the property for $2.2 million with the understanding that proceeds of future land sales would be shared with the state. The town of Westborough put the remaining 37-acre parcel up for sale in 2016. A full request for proposals was released, and potential bidders were given a tour of the buildings in July. When no viable proposals were received, the deadline for the sale was extended to October 5. The winning proposal came from Pulte Homes who proposed a 700-unit housing development for seniors who are 55 or over. (Courtesy Michael Martin and Matt Keefe.)

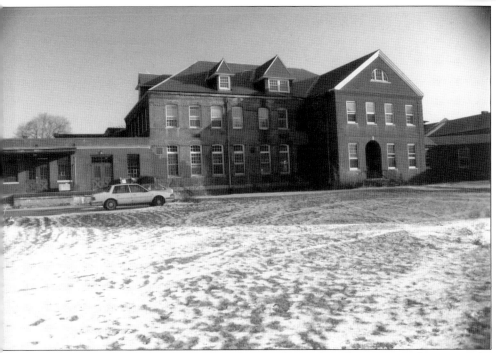

While the congregate dining model continued at Westborough well into the 20th century, the hospital eventually outgrew the original dining hall in the administration building when the overall census exceeded 2,000 patients. In 1933, a larger, more modern dining facility was added to the left rear of the administration building and connected to it and the wards by hallways. The kitchen housed a large dining hall, staff cafeterias, the bakery, and cold storage. Large banks of ovens, industrial mixing hardware, and the original cafeteria line remain in the cafeteria along with a collection of broken dishes and trays. (Above, courtesy National Register of Historic Places; below, courtesy Daimon Paul.)

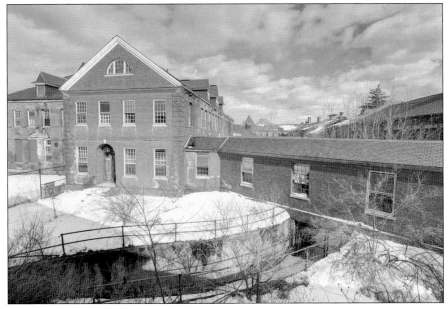

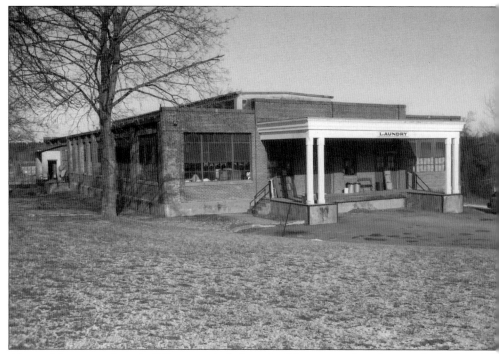

Along with a spate of new buildings, particularly outbuildings, a new laundry was also built in 193
and stayed in use until the hospital's closing. In the early years, patients were responsible for a
the laundry and mending on campus, but also took in a good deal of work for other institution:
There were other laundry facilities located in the farm colonies, but they were no longer in us
by the early 1960s. Water was piped directly from the water tower to the laundry building, an
once the electricity was carried out to the building, the wooden hand washers were replaced wit
electric ones. These machines are the only remaining fixtures in the laundry. (Above, courtes
National Register of Historic Places; below, courtesy Diane Danthony.)

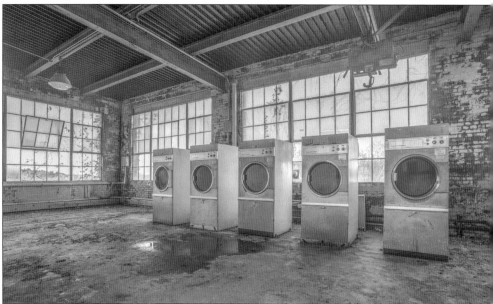

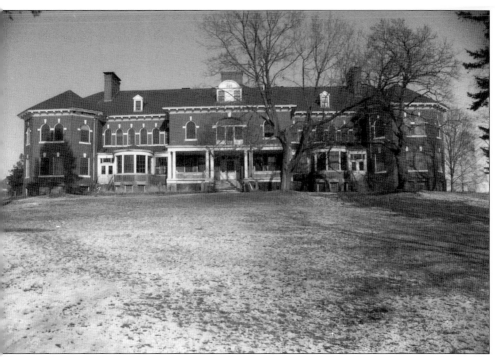

In later years, a number of fires were reported on campus. In 1971, a fire broke out in the linen room of the Talbot Building. By then, the building was being used as a rehabilitation center for long-term patients who were being transitioned back into the community. The program was controversial, as many believed that long-term patients could not be returned to society. The building's elegant mantle pieces have either disappeared or been vandalized, and the day rooms are now filled with discarded patient beds and furniture. The round brick porches have collapsed, and a fence surrounds the building. (Above, courtesy National Register of Historic Places; below, courtesy Michael Martin and Matt Keefe.)

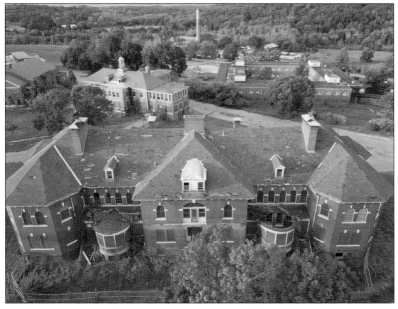

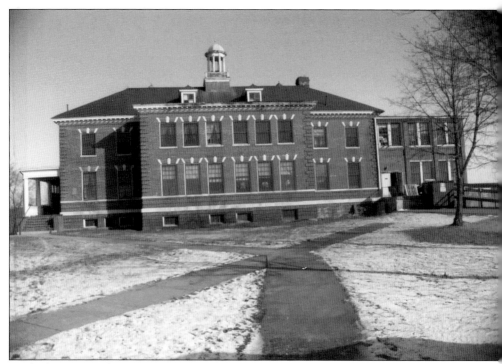

By the late 1960s, the wards in both wings of the Codman Building had been consolidated into smaller programs within the building, mirroring the unitization of the main hospital building. The printing shop in the basement continued to produce the patient newsletter called *Chatter Chips*. For a time, Codman was used as an admissions building rather than as patient wards, sitting vacant for a few weeks at a time between shifts in usage. The ornate sunporch was boxed in at some point, and a garage door was added where there were once windows. The building is now used occasionally for law enforcement training. It was demolished in 2019. (Above, courtesy National Register of Historic Places; below, courtesy Diane Danthony.)

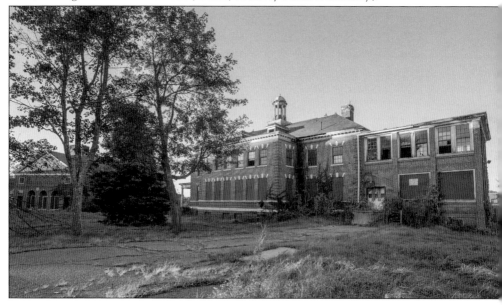

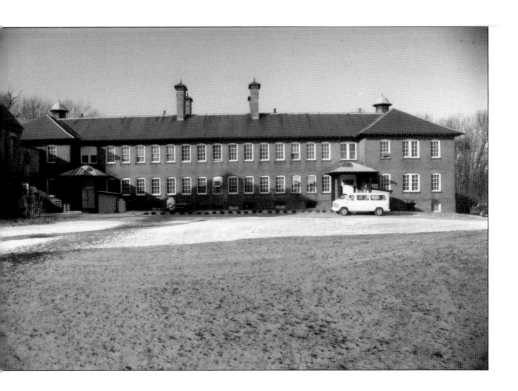

uilt in 1906, hospital Wards I and J sit off to the left of the main hospital facing Wards G and I and housed male patients. The two-story brick building was a plain, symmetrical building with pen-air porches to the rear that overlooked the hospital's corn fields. Later, this building would ouse the Robert F. Kennedy Children's Action Corps, a residential treatment facility for juvenile ffenders. The program would eventually move into the former Paine Hall, where it would remain or a number of years until the building was taken over by the Massachusetts Department of Youth ervices. (Above, courtesy National Register of Historic Places; below, courtesy Jennifer Engle.)

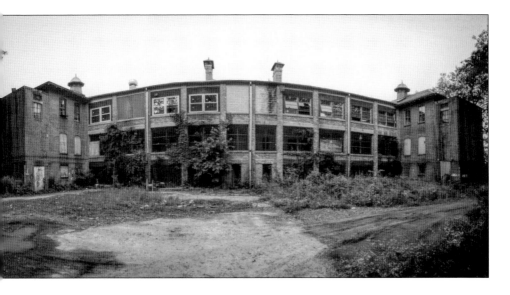

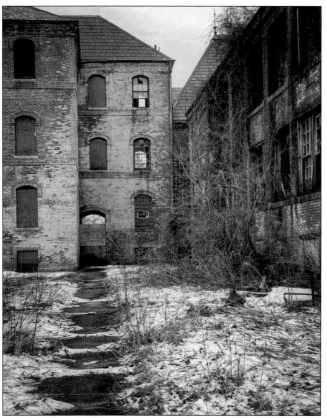

As the hospital was added onto in the early 20th centur a number of courtyards and passageways were created by the connecting hallways and can still be seen today. Though inaccessible from the road, it is possible to see into some of the interior courtyards as well as where picnic pavilions were in use until the hospital's closure in 2010. After a number of fires in the female wards, as well as a massive hole in the roof, the middle of the female ward collapsed completely. The collapsed portion of the building was being used for storage, and debris is now mixed with filin cabinets, desks, and chairs. (Courtesy Jennifer Engle.)

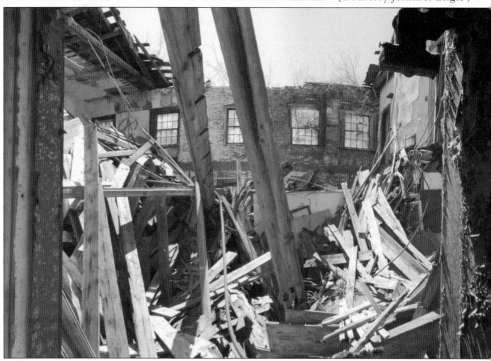

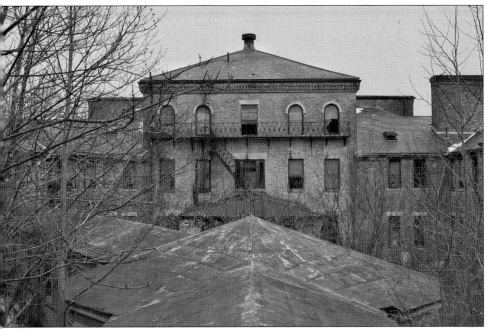

timately, a 15-member panel was largely responsible for the closing of Westborough State
ospital. The money saved from the early closure of the hospital would be reallocated to community
acement services, presumably allowing the hospital a greater level of resources in discharging
tients. Earlier in 2009, the demolition of several buildings on the hospital campus was included
a state list of "shovel ready" projects to be funded by a federal stimulus package. The cost of the
molition was estimated to be $4.9 million. The report also recommended that the state close a
-bed inpatient unit at Quincy Mental Health Center and decrease inpatient beds at Tewksbury
ate Hospital. (Above, courtesy Matt Keefe; below, courtesy Diane Danthony.)

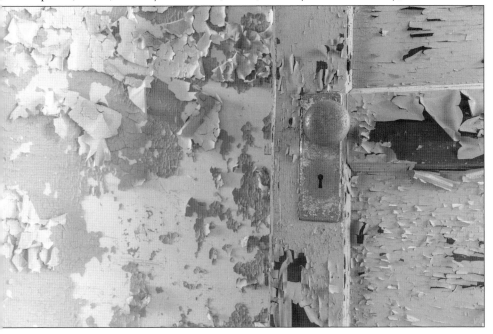

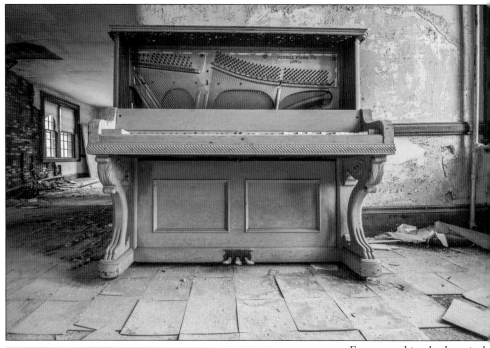

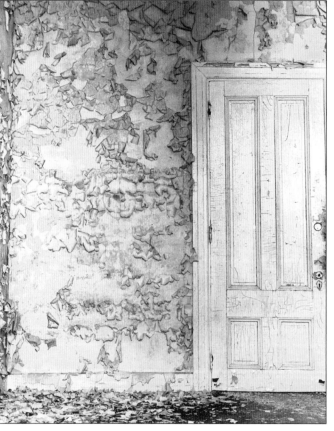

Every ward in the hospital, both in the main building and in the smaller hospital buildings, were furnished with at least one piano. A number of these pianos remain, as well as furniture, linens, and medical equipment. There are boxes of Christmas decorations as well as art supplies and, often, books scattered throughout. Ther is furniture and medical equipment strewn across th lawns, having been remove from the buildings and discarded. Exposure to the elements has heightened th level of decay inside and ha made the buildings unsafe in spite of the relatively unchanged exteriors of the hospital. (Above, courtesy Brian Pawlowskis; below, courtesy Jennifer Engle.)

When Westborough was in operation, fire was a constant concern, and a number of measures were taken over the years to keep on top of fire safety. However, once the buildings were left vacant, the risk of fire grew far greater as the buildings were left unattended and vulnerable to arson. On June 3, 2018, shortly before the first demolition announcement would be made, a two-alarm fire broke out in Ward A. The female ward, already collapsed and badly damaged, was further damaged by the fire that was quickly extinguished by the Westborough Fire Department. The fire was investigated, but the source of the blaze was not determined. (Right, courtesy Westborough Fire Department; below, courtesy Jennifer Engle.)

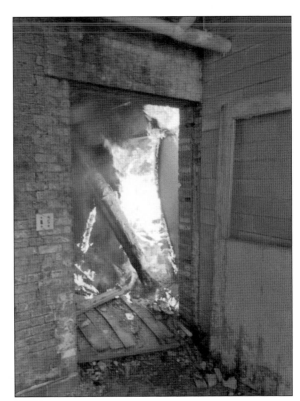

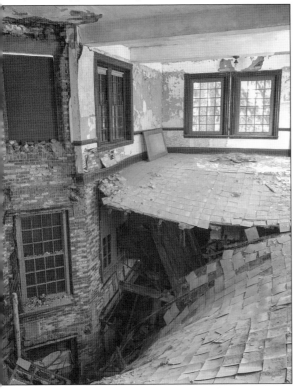

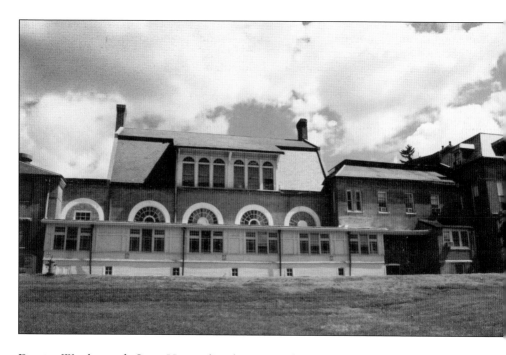

Despite Westborough State Hospital's relative popularity with photographers and historian there was no concerted effort to preserve any of the original campus as there was at Danve State Hospital and Northampton State Hospital (both built on the well-known Kirkbride Plan The future of the still active Department of Youth Services buildings remains unclear, as th main campus is fenced off and readied for abatement. As of the writing of this book, only th main administration building remains standing. (Above, courtesy Massachusetts Department ⟨ Mental Health; below, courtesy Diane Danthony.)

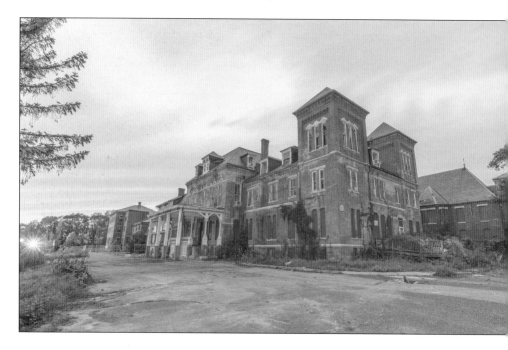